THE DIAGNOSIS AND TREATMENT

OF

SPEECH AND READING PROBLEMS

(Tenth Printing)

THE DIAGNOSIS AND TREATMENT

OF

SPEECH AND READING PROBLEMS

By

CARL H. DELACATO, Ed.D.

Director

The Developmental Reading Program
Chestnut Hill Academy

Psychological Services
The Rehabilitation Center

The Chestnut Hill Reading Clinic

The Institute of Language Disability

Philadelphia, Pennsylvania

Illustrations by

Mary Lee Lowry

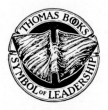

CHARLES C THOMAS · PUBLISHER
Springfield · Illinois · U. S. A.

Published and Distributed Throughout the World by

CHARLES C THOMAS · PUBLISHER

BANNERSTONE HOUSE

301-327 East Lawrence Avenue, Springfield, Illinois, U.S.A.

NATCHEZ PLANTATION HOUSE

735 North Atlantic Boulevard, Fort Lauderdale, Florida, U.S.A.

First Printing, 1963, 2000 copies
Second Printing, 1964, 2000 copies
Third Printing, 1964, 2000 copies
Fourth Printing, 1965, 2000 copies
Fifth Printing, 1965, 2000 copies
Sixth Printing, December, 1965, 2000 copies
Seventh Printing, May, 1966, 2000 copies
Eighth Printing, March, 1967, 3000 copies
Ninth Printing, January, 1968, 3000 copies
Tenth Printing, January, 1970, 3000 copies

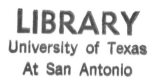
Printed in the United States of America
H-2

To

Liz, Hank and David

For what they have taught me of the mysteries of human development and to their Uncle Glenn *who is Glenn Doman, Director of The Rehabilitation Center at Philadelphia, whose creative insights and hard work have given to the world of science many new concepts and procedures in the field of clinical and developmental neurology.*

ACKNOWLEDGMENTS

I wish to thank those many physicians, nurses, teachers, psychologists, and therapists who have helped to create, to criticize and to refine the conceptual basis of the neuro-psychological approach to language and reading problems. To those too numerous to mention fellow workers in the field from all over the country who reacted to *The Treatment and Prevention of Reading Problems* in the way in which I hoped—by research, I am very grateful. For the volumes of research material forwarded to me or published—all of which have helped to crystalize the problems which we have not solved, and have helped to clarify immeasurably my original statement of the concept of *Neurological Organization,* I am also very appreciative.

I am grateful to the following men and the institutions which they represent for their great help, for these men and their institutions made possible most of the research referred to in this book: Dr. Eugene Spitz, Chief of Pediatric Neurosurgery, Children's Hospital, Philadelphia; Dr. Robert Doman, Medical Director, The Rehabilitation Center at Philadelphia; the late Mr. George Hamilton, President, Keystone View Company, Meadville, Pa.; Mr. J. Harrison Worrall, Assistant Director, The Chestnut Hill Reading Clinic, Philadelphia; Mr. Robert Kingsley, Headmaster, Chestnut Hill Academy, Philadelphia; Mr. James Wolf, Director, Special Education, Panama Canal Zone; and Dr. Raymundo Veras, Director, Centro de Rehabilitacoa, Rio de Janeiro, Brazil.

I am indebted to the following co-workers at The Rehabilitation Center at Philadelphia: Col. Anthony Flores, Dr. Edward Le Winn, Dr. Sidney Greenstein, the late Dr. Sigmund Le Winn, Rosemary Warnock, Florence Sharp, Lindley Boyer, Charles Burhns, John Tini, Takako Suzuki, Greta Erdtmann, Lorraine Forrest and Andrew DeLuca.

To my co-workers at the Chestnut Hill Reading Clinic: Daniel

W. Charles, Susanne Van Nolde, Laine Santa Maria, David M. Rutter, Dr. Ben Lubin, Dr. Russell Sinoway, and to Dr. Donald Blake who is in great part responsible for Chapter 4, I am very grateful.

The author is deeply indebted to these classroom teachers who were courageous enough to listen to a new concept in education and to use these concepts in their classrooms: Elizabeth Anderson, Nancy Brewer, Elisabeth Carnwath, Helen Coates, Albert Conkey, Barbara Crawford, Betty Cressman, Richard Cutler, Mary Dee, Alexander Dowbenko, Melvyn Ehrlich, Virginia Engels, Sallyanne Hansell, Madeline Harper, Patricia Inch, William Kershaw, Edward Lawless, Amelia Lodge, George Miller, John Miller, John Morford, William Phelps, Henry Putsch, Stanley Robinson, Katherine Roper, Susan Santa Maria, Francis Steel, Anne Swain, Jeanne Tucker, Mrs. Albert Tyler, Percy Wales, Perot Walker, Elizabeth Walker, Horace Witman, Theodore Wright and Diane Zacherle. These teachers made possible the first practical applications of these concepts in normal classroom situations. Without their willingness to try something new, and therefore strange to teachers, students and parents, these concepts would still remain untried and unproved theories.

I wish to thank Francis Steel and E. B. Gilchrist, Jr. for the photographs. I wish to thank Mary Lee Lowry for the illustrations. I am most indebted to my secretary, Anne Eggleton, for her great help in collecting and collating data and her help in preparing this manuscript.

Finally, I am most indebted to Janice, my wife, for her constant help, understanding and encouragement.

C. H. D.

CONTENTS

Page

Acknowledgments vii

Chapter

1. Neurological Organization: Concept 3
2. The Nature of Language Problems 8
3. An Historical Overview of the Problem 14
4. The Phylogeny of Neurological Organization 26
      Environmental Forces 27
      Medulla and Spinal Cord 35
      Pons 37
      Mid-brain 39
      Cortex 40
      Cortical Hemispheric Dominance 41
5. The Ontogeny of Neurological Organization 47
      Medulla and Spinal Cord 48
      Pons 49
      Mid-brain 52
      Cortex 56
      Cortical Hemispheric Dominance 63
6. Neurological Organization and Brain Injury 68
7. Diagnostic Procedures 79
      Medulla and Spinal Cord 85
      Pons 86
      Mid-brain 87
      Cortex 88
      Cortical Hemispheric Dominance 90
8. Treatment Procedures 102
      Medulla and Spinal Cord 104
      Pons 105
      Mid-brain 110

Page

Chapter

Cortex 113
Cortical Hemispheric Dominance 122
9. Case Materials 136

Bibliography 176
Index 183

THE DIAGNOSIS AND TREATMENT

OF

SPEECH AND READING PROBLEMS

Chapter 1

NEUROLOGICAL ORGANIZATION: CONCEPT

PREREQUISITE to the reading of this book is the reading of *The Treatment and Prevention of Reading Problems* which is the author's original statement of the neuro-psychological approach to the development of language and of the concept of *Neurological Organization.*

The concepts contained in the following pages are the result of the collection of data in testing the hypotheses proposed in *The Treatment and Prevention of Reading Problems.* Some of those concepts are changed, a few are negated, and most are made stronger. It remains a valid statement of the basic premises of the neuro-psychological approach to language and reading problems. This book is in essence an addendum to *The Treatment and Prevention of Reading Problems.* It is the product of much research. The subjects used were 600 severely brain injured children, 500 brain injured adults, 100 post operative neurological patients, 200 now deceased laboratory rabbits, 600 normal children with speech and/or reading problems, and 800 children who presented no problem of movement or communication. Many co-workers were required to carry out our studies.

The design was simple. We theorized, experimented, collected and evaluated results and then re-theorized. Our basic criterion was, "Are we getting results?" We carefully avoided the modern dilemma described by Dr. William Brownell in his address to the American Educational Research Association in Atlantic City, New Jersey on February 15, 1960.

".... What I am speaking for, I suppose, is research in depth as contrasted with research in which shallowness is hidden be-

[3]

neath a surface of technical excellence; for research characterized by logical analysis, shrewd insight and sagacious fore-
sight as contrasted with that amounting to little more than the
shuffling of numbers; for research undertaken only after much
sweat, prayer and profanity have been expended upon the
problem in all its ramifications.

I have chosen to emphasize the merits of simple research
designs because they enable us to concentrate on our problem
and on what it entails by way of significant data and procedures for procuring them. When we engage in such research,
we need not fear lest we be charged with being unscientific.
There is nothing in the concept of scientific method to justify
collecting and relying upon trivial evidence, no matter how
impressive its volume or how involved the treatment accorded
it. . . . .[1]

The author made the original statement of Neurological Organization in *The Treatment and Prevention of Reading Problems* in 1959. In the original the author wrote:

"Neurological organization is that physiologically optimum condition which exists uniquely and most completely in man and
is the result of a total and uninterrupted ontogenetic neural
development. This development recapitulates the phylogenetic
neural development of man and begins during the first tri-
mester of gestation and ends at about six and one half years
of age in normal humans. This orderly development in humans
progresses vertically through the spinal cord and all other areas
of the central nervous system up to the level of the cortex, as
it does with all mammals. Man's final and unique developmental progression takes place at the level of the cortex and it
is lateral (from left to right or from right to left).

"This progression is an interdependent continuum, hence if
a high level of development is unfunctioning or incomplete,
such as in sleep or as the result of trauma, lower levels become
operative and dominant (mid-brain sleep and high cervical
pathological reflexes). If a lower level is incomplete, all suc-
ceeding higher levels are affected both in relation to their

---

[1]Brownell, William A.: Research in the Decade Ahead, Address at the Annual
Banquet, American Educational Research Association, Atlantic City, New Jersey,
February 15, 1960, page 3.

height in the central nervous system and in relation to the chronology of their development. Man's only contribution to this organizational schema is that he has added to the vertical progression, the final lateral progression at the level of the cortex. Here again, at the cortical level, the same premises apply. The final progression must become dominant and must

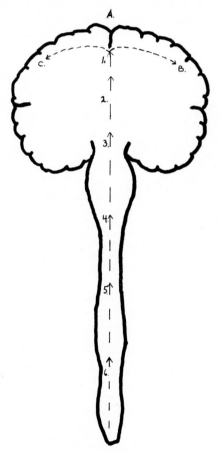

Figure 1. Neuro-organizational schema (posterior view). A. The point to which animals slightly lower phylogenetically than man can arrive. B. Point to which totally developed left-sided human arrives. C. Point to which totally developed right-sided human arrives. Numbers denote lower neural levels which affect higher levels and which are in turn affected by higher levels. Upon failure of a higher level next lower level becomes dominant.

(Courtesy Charles C Thomas, Publisher, Springfield, Illinois.)

supersede all others. Prerequisite, however, to such dominance
is the adequate development of all lower levels.

In totally developed man the left or the right cortical hemisphere must become dominant, with lower prerequisite requirements met, if his organization is to be complete (see
Fig. 1).

"Phylogenetics is the study of the evolution of man. Phylogenetically the nervous system has evolved from a very simple
to a very complex mechanism. As evolution progressed, animals achieved what could be compared to a spinal cord. These
animals operated chiefly at a reflex level. As time went on in the
evolutionary cycle, the mid-brain was developed, and finally
there evolved animals which operated slightly under the level
of man, who has a cortex. Through the evolutionary cycle man
has developed a cortex, yet vestigially he retains the lower
level neurological appendages and functions which were
needed during this developmental cycle. If the animals which
operate slightly under the level of man are analyzed, they are
found to have a cortex. Generally, they have the neuro-
anatomical structure of man but these animals cannot do the
following things: stand fully upright, see three-dimensionally,
oppose the thumb and forefinger, supinate and pronate the
hand, speak or write a language and, operate unilaterally with
hand, foot and eye of one side of the body.

"The neurological differences between man and slightly lower
forms of animals are not cellularly important. The basic difference between man and the animal world is that man has
achieved cortical dominance wherein one side of the cortex
controls the skills in which man outdistances lower forms of
animals. This whole phylogenetic process is recapitulated ontogenetically with each human being. In the event that there is
some obstruction to this ontogenetic recapitulation, communication and language dysfunctions occur.

"Man has evolved to the point that the two hemispheres of
the brain, although they mirror each other physically, have
differentiated functions. Right handed humans are one sided,
i.e., they are right eyed, right footed and right handed, with
the left cortical hemisphere controlling the organism.

"Trauma of the controlling cortical hemisphere results in loss
of language skills, but equally important, trauma of the sub-

dominant area results in loss of tonal factors. Left hemiplegics (right handed people who have suffered a cerebrovascular accident to the right or subdominant hemisphere of the cortex) have no difficulty with speech but suffer a very significant loss in tonal memory, tonal appreciation and the ability to carry a tune. Generally, their melody, rhythm and accent abilities are affected.

"Some investigators feel that man's supremacy is not the result of cellular acquisitions within the cortex but is instead the result of the specialization of function which man has evolved in the use of his cortex. They feel that as man evolved into an ideating and communicating human being, he simultaneously developed cortical laterality."[2]

The basic premise of the neuro-psychological approach as outlined by the author is that if man does not follow this schema he exhibits a problem of mobility or communication. To overcome such problems one evaluates the subject via the neurological schema outlined above. Those areas of neurological organization which have not been completed or are absent are overcome by *passively imposing* them upon the nervous system in those with problems of mobility and are *taught* to those with problems of speech or reading. When the neurological organization is complete the problem is overcome.

Since speech and reading are uniquely human, we have focalized upon them in our efforts to educate our children. Speech and reading are the final *human* result of neurological organization and hence are clinical indices of the nature and the quality of neurological organization of an individual.

[2]Delacato, C. H.: *The Treatment and Prevention of Reading Problems,* Springfield, Thomas, 1959, pp. 19-22.

Chapter 2

THE NATURE OF LANGUAGE PROBLEMS

Educators and therapists have historically categorized language and reading problems symptomatically. The groups treating these problems have named themselves and have set up criteria for licensure in many states within this symptomatic orientation. Such problems have not only been categorized symptomatically, diagnosed symptomatically, but have also been treated symptomatically and therefore unsuccessfully. The language problems listed below are the usual list one finds—as the different problems of speech and reading. They are treated by personnel with backgrounds of training varying with the problem. *They are not separate problems—they are simply varying degrees of the same problem—therefore have the same cause and need the same treatment—the only variable being one of degree.*

Let us list the problems as they usually appear:
1. Aphasia
2. Delayed Speech
3. Stuttering
4. Retarded Reading
5. Poor Spelling and Handwriting
6. Reading which falls within normal range but is below Mathematical Performance.

These are six degrees of communication dysfunction. If we are to deal with language dysfunction successfully, we must be cognizant of this relationship. In the past we have organized educative services and re-educative services from this symptomatic bias. We have, therefore, been unable to diagnose these problems causally or to treat them causally. We have gone into six blind alleys in search of peripheral answers, not seeing that they were all aspects of the same problem. Let us look at the problems as they exist.

APHASIA

Aphasia is the name given to speech and reading retardation when there is suspected brain damage. These children are usually treated as if the problem is with the lips, tongue, and larynx. One can immediately see the lack of logic in defining the problem as brain damage and treating it as mouth and throat damage.

These children have an over-all problem of communication. Speech and reading are only small parts of their communication problem. They have perceptual distortions and conceptual distortions. Their inability to communicate is so basic as to distort their gestural behavior which does not require speech—indeed, they have great difficulty relating to others at a body image level. They have great difficulty communicating their feelings adequately. They even have great difficulty communicating empathy—one of our most basic communication modalities. This is a severe language dysfunction. The other problems are the same but are less severe.

DELAYED OR POORLY ARTICULATED SPEECH

This group shows a retardation in the development of word concepts, saying single words and sentences. This group is usually seen in speech clinics at about the age of three. It is one of the most difficult groups to diagnose. Where there is speech but where it is delayed, the problem becomes a real problem to the schools dealing with children of four and one-half to six. At this point these children, who are in essence delayed in speech, present a picture of immature speech and poor articulation. Historically we have concerned ourselves with the emotional status and the auditory discrimination of this group—*completely peripheral approaches.*

These children are delayed neurologically as a rule, and the delayed speech is only one facet of the neurological delay. We invariably find them delayed in many areas with their basic delay lying in poor neurological organization.

STUTTERING

Historically we have been concerned with the speech of stutterers. Stutterers stutter in many areas. They stutter in speech—they stutter visually—they stutter in mobility—they stutter auditorially—and they stutter manually. We have treated them as if they merely stuttered in speech. They stutter in these many areas because they have not developed a dominant cortical hemisphere. They can't stutter when we make one hemisphere dominant (such as when we ask them to sing). We have all seen pencil stutterers, indeed it is easily observed that when a stutterer is writing or tracing over a figure with a pencil and begins to stutter in his speech he also begins to stutter in his writing. Stutterers have been treated as if they had only one problem and as if that problem was always found in the mouth or throat.

RETARDED READING

This group begins to be recognized with low reading readiness scores and its symptomatology becomes immediately evident with beginning reading.

"The reading pattern of these children showed a very early and consistent history in grades one and two of reversals, that is, reading and writing words such as *was* for *saw*, *on* for *no*, reading and writing numbers such as 24 for 42. These same children were very poor in early spelling and, if they were fair readers at the time still tended to be poor spellers, reversing letters within words periodically. We found in the reading pattern indications of great difficulty with the word sight method and, when the method was changed, equally slow mastery of the alphabet or phonetic system. We also found that at all ages these children tended to have higher vocabulary scores than comprehension scores on standardized tests and their reading speed seemed to be very slow. They tended to have significantly more difficulty during early reading years with small words than with large words. Generally they disliked reading. They seemed unable to associate symbols, be they words or sounds, with ideas. They also tended to be good in other academic areas, especially the area of arithmetic. They tended at the secondary school level to have much higher mathematical ability scores than language ability scores on tests of scholastic aptitude. They tended as they went through the junior high and secondary school years to have low marks in English and most of their reading courses, but tended to do well in memory courses and courses involving mathematics and mechanical skills."[1]

POOR SPELLING AND HANDWRITING

This group many times reads passably. The poor spellers tend to reverse letters within words instead of reversing whole words as the poor readers do. If a child in this group studies a list of words for a spelling test, he usually does quite well on the test but if asked to spell the same words 3 days later he fails miserably. Teaching such children spelling is a waste of time for student, teacher, and usually parent until the child is neurologically organized.

Poor writers have two significant characteristics. Their handwriting is disorganized, i.e. there is great variation in the size of the letters and in the spacing between letters and words. They also tend to tilt their heads strangely when writing, tend to assume strange sitting positions or move their heads constantly while writing.

READING PERFORMANCE AND APTITUDES WHICH FALL WITHIN THE NORMAL RANGE BUT WHICH ARE LOWER THAN MATHEMATICAL SCORES AND APTITUDES

This group is characterized in adulthood by becoming engineers, mathematicians, and technical scientists. Many of these men are extremely bright and have above average language and reading performance. Their mathematical ability, however, is significantly higher than their verbal ability. Too often this group chooses its vocational bias through default. A mild lack of neurological organization is present, and as a result the path

---

[1]Delacato, C.: *The Treatment and Prevention of Reading Problems*, Springfield, Thomas, 1959, pp. 8 and 9.

of least resistance is chosen. Through neurological organization the verbal performance of this group could be improved to a point more in keeping with the mathematical score.

These six categories have been treated as six different anomalies. When we view a child ontogenetically we see the same six areas occur in the developmental process toward good communication.

The newborn has all of the symptoms of the aphasic child. He has a total inability to communicate other than by crying. As he develops he begins to communicate on a sound and gestural level—without words just as does the child with delayed speech. When he reaches the age of three and has progressed neurologically to the point where early choices of laterality are being made, he goes through a very natural phase of indecision and stuttering. As he moves through this neurological stage, he becomes lateralized and then depending on the degree of lateralization he reads, spells, writes and develops those skills which in the aggregate represent verbal aptitude and verbal performance.

Children who are being treated successfully for one of the six problems described above must move from one level to the next if they are to achieve complete communication function.

Reading Below Mathematical Performance

Poor Spelling and Handwriting

Retarded Reading

Stuttering

Delayed Speech

Aphasia

As a child in any one of these categories shows progress, he naturally moves into the next category.

The aphasic goes into delayed speech.

Delayed speech goes into stuttering.

Stuttering goes into poor reading.

Poor reading goes into poor spelling and writing.

Poor spelling and writing go into lower verbal performance and aptitude than mathematical aptitude.

Those children who are older and therefore are more difficult to move through these natural developmental stages, are our failures. For example, a stutterer who has been taught to read while his speech remains at the three year level (stuttering) is the tragic result of our peripheral categorization and treatment. Such children, who are bright, become mathematicians and scientists by default, for by not treating the communication problem we have left them verbally disabled in language. As a result they can never reach their true potential in the area of communication.

In this book we are discussing all of these problems. Those with severe lacks of neurological organization have severe symptoms such as aphasia. Those with very mild lacks of neurological organization have reading and writing scores which fall within normal limits but below their mathematical performance. The difference is merely one of degree.

Chapter 3

AN HISTORICAL OVERVIEW OF THE PROBLEM

Ever since men have suspected that there was a relationship between the nervous system and language function, we have fallen into two great errors:

1. *We have equated handedness with cortical hemispheric dominance.* Obviously, handedness is only one single aspect of many which indicate cortical hemispheric dominance. As a result of this error we have never searched deeply enough into the clinical indices of cortical hemispheric dominance, indeed, as a result of this error, we have never made a valid effort to define, "cortical hemispheric dominance."

2. *We have equated cerebral dominance (which we have not defined) with neurological maturity.*

The literature abounds with these two great errors. No researcher has given us data as to the reliability of any of our tests of cortical hemispheric dominance. We have naively accepted the hand with which the patient writes as the valid and complete indication of his hemispheric dominance. We know that this is not a valid test, indeed, it is not even a reliable test.

If we accept the lack of sophistication involved in equating handedness alone to hemispheric dominance, we are negating a vast store of neurological data. We know, for instance, that if we ask a completely right sided human being to write by holding a pencil in his toes and writing by moving his foot, that he will be able to write with his right foot but will not be able to write with his left foot. Using the naive rationale of equating a single factor to hemispheric dominance we could, therefore, have an infinitely more reliable and more valid test of hemispheric dominance if we gave the patient a pencil and asked him to remove his shoes and to write his name and address with his feet. This would certainly seem more valid than using the hand as the sole criterion for hemispheric dominance, for very few people are actually taught to write with their feet and the test would not be biased by cultural and educational variations.

Using the single unreliable criterion of hand choice as the indication of hemispheric dominance we have then proceeded to equate this with complete neurological maturation. We have done this while ignoring the wealth of experimental and clinical data which we have on the phylogenesis and the ontogenesis of the human nervous system.

These errors were initiated in the earliest writings of men who had theories on the relationship of handedness and human function. Plato, Carlyle and Lombrosa helped to start us down this erroneous path.[1]

Even our present leaders in the field perpetuate these errors. Men such as Zangwill tend to equate the mere ascertainment of handedness as the significant criterion of hemispheric dominance. They follow with the implication that cortical hemispheric dominance is, in fact, the prime criterion for neurological maturity.[2]

This is not only true for the leaders in the field but is also true for those other workers in the field who, on the basis of such data, naively but strongly state that these factors are, therefore, not significantly related to language problems.[3]

Broca and Jackson gave impetus to the tendency to equate handedness with neurological sufficiency through their writings which were the earliest containing physiological data.[4, 5]

[1]Blau, A.: *The Master Hand*, New York, The American Orthopsychiatric Association, Inc., 1946, 5, pp. 1-206.

[2]Zangwill, O. L.: *Cerebral Dominance and its Relation to Psychological Function*, Edinburgh, Oliver and Boyd, 1960, pp. 1-31.

[3]Money, J.: *Reading Disability, Progress and Research Needs in Dyslexia*, Baltimore, Johns Hopkins Press, 1962, pp. 1-222.

[4]Broca, P.: *Memoirs Sur Le Creveau de l'Homme*, Paris, C. Reinwald, 1888, pp. 1-161.

[5]Jackson, J. H.: Observations on the Physiology of Language, London, *Med. Times and Gaz.*, 2:275; Reprinted in *Brain*, 38:59-64, 1915.

One can see the immediate reaction to these pioneers and their work by looking at the literature of the times. Handedness became strongly entrenched as the sole criterion of cortical hemispheric dominance.[6, 7, 8, 9]

As one can readily see, these early papers equating handedness with cortical hemispheric dominance and relating them to speech generally appeared in the Journals of Great Britain. There followed a great number of such articles in the Journals of Great Britain, most of which tended to perpetuate the errors. Even today, the literature of Great Britain persists in this bias.[10, 11, 12, 13, 14]

The beginning of the twentieth century in the United States found one group searching in vain to correlate handedness with language function. Others worked with slightly different biases.[15, 16]

These men hoped to find how handedness or hemispheric dominance asserts itself in humans.

[6]Jackson, J. H.: Defect of Intellectual Expression (Aphasia) with Left Hemiplegia, *Lancet*, 1: 457, 1868.

[7]Dally: Observation D'aphasie Avec Hemiplegie Gauche, *Ann. Med. Psychol., Paris*, 8:252-253, 1882.

[8]Bateman, F.: On Aphasia and The Localization of the Faculty of Speech, *Med. Times and Gaz.*, pp. 486-488; 540-542, 1869.

[9]Bramwell, B.: On "Crossed" Aphasia and the factors which go to determine whether the "Leading" or "Driving" Speech-centers shall be located in the left or the right hemisphere of the brain. With notes on a case of "Crossed" aphasia (Aphasia with right-sided hemiplegia) in a left-handed man, *Lancet*, 1:1473-1479, 1899.

[10]Brain, W. R.: Speech and Handedness, *Lancet*, 2:837-842, 1945.

[11]Brain, W. R.: Aphasia, Apraxia and Agnosia, in Wilson, K., *Neurology*, London, Butterworth, III, pp. 1413-1483, 1955.

[12]Clark, M. N.: *Left-Handedness; Laterality Characteristics and Their Educational Implications*, London, University of London Press, 1957.

[13]Ettlinger, G., Jackson, C. F., and Zangwill, O. L.: Cerebral Dominance, in Sinistrals, *Brain*, 79:569-588, 1956.

[14]Goodglass, H. and Quadfasel, F. A.: Language Laterality in Left-handed Patients, *Brain*, 77:521-548, 1954.

[15]Newman, R.: The Question of Mirror-Imaging in Human One-Egg Twins, *Human Biol.*, 12:21, 1940.

[16]Veeler, S.: On The Amount of External Mirror-Imagery in Double Monsters and Identical Twins, *Proc. Nat. Acad., Sci.*, 15:839, 1929.

Others used sociological data to ascertain whether cultural and educational experiences influenced sidedness or the expression of sidedness.[17, 18]

There was little progress until Samuel Orton again attacked the problem armed with more neurological data which we had garnered from our experience in World War I.

Dr. Samuel T. Orton revived the concept during the modern era. In his writings he described a diagnostic rationale which evaluated the level of cortical hemispheric dominance. His contributions in this field were widely recognized. There were for a considerable length of time many followers of the Orton rationale. By the late 1930's this following began to diminish and the neurological approach to language fell into disuse among educators.[19]

The author feels that this was the unfortunate result of a lack of real understanding of the neurological basis of language and its development by Orton and his followers. Orton was a brilliant and pioneering neurologist who moved back the frontier of diagnostic knowledge in his field. True, we now have another half century of research in the field of neurology and the development of functional neurology from its infancy to help us diagnostically, but we must recognize the contribution made by Orton. Unhappily, Orton fell prey to the educational bias of the times and postulated treatment in a field which was new to him and which was unrelated to his diagnostic rationale. The lack of logic taken by his followers was in great part responsible for the lack of progress in this area. His followers convinced him that teaching children phonetics would in great part overcome neurological difficulties. This is obviously treating the symptom and is completely unrelated to the cause.

Teaching children phonetics is productive of results with those few children who have not been taught phonetics. It is

---

[17]Jensen, B. T.: Left-Right Orientation in Profile Drawing, *Amer. Journ. of Psychol.*, LXV:80-83, Jan., 1952.

[18]Jensen, B. T., Reading Habits and Left-Right Orientation in Profile Drawing by Japanese Children, *Amer. Journ. of Psychol.*, LXV, pp. 306-307, April, 1952.

[19]Orton, S. T.: *Reading, Writing and Speech Problems in Children*, New York, W. W. Norton Co., 1937, pp. 1-215.

much more realistic and much more productive of results if we treat children who have been diagnosed as having a neurological etiology relative to their poor reading, *neurologically*. The untenable position taken by the followers of Orton was that they were merely treating symptoms and that, although they had learned to diagnose the etiology, the treatment was unrelated.

It is obvious that, if the problem lies in the nervous system, we must treat the nervous system.

As a result of the unfortunate bias given to Orton's diagnostic concepts, the research in the field has lagged. The search for new knowledge continued in the field of neurology while the field of reading and speech teaching went off into many tangents of technique, seeming always to neglect the mainstream of potential answers.

As Gesell *et al.* began to investigate and to write, the first trace of a wholistic and developmental rationale became evident.[20]

These workers looked at a human being from birth on and began to gain insights of a developmental nature. They began to see that handedness was a developmental phenomenon and that there were many other indices of neurological maturation in addition to handedness.

From this work sprang a new developmental school of thought relative to vision, known as the Optometric Extension Program, with leaders such as Skeffington, Harmon and Getman.[21, 22, 23]

This school of thought sees the organisms' relationship to vision developmentally. They feel that man must learn to see and that his vision depends upon his mobility, experience and the world he lives in. This group, which sprang from Gesell, represents a dynamic approach to the ontogentic development of hu-

[20]Gesell, A., Ilg, F., And Bullis, G.: *Vision: Its Development in Infant and Child*, New York, Paul B. Hoebner Inc., 1950.

[21]Harmon, D. B.: *Notes on a Dynamic Theory of Vision*, pub. by the author, Austin, Texas, 1958.

[22]Getman, G.: *How to Develop Your Child's Intelligence*, pub. by the author, Luverne, Minn., 1959.

[23]Skeffington, A. M.: *Differential Diagnosis in Ocular Examination*, Chicago, Wilton Pub. Co., 1931, pp. 1-200.

man vision as it relates to neurological maturation. Both their diagnostic and treatment rationales for visual problems are based upon developmental concepts.

Some workers began to investigate the possibility that the function of the two hemispheres operating in concert via sub-cortical means was significant. By investigating the function of the corpus callosum, which lies immediately under the cortex, they found that indeed there were many areas of function where the two hemispheres interacted reciprocally via sub-cortical means. These men found that there was a significant relationship of sub-cortical function to what was generally clinically ascribed to the cortex. They also found many areas of function which were interhemispherically controlled.[24, 25, 26, 27, 28, 29, 30, 31]

Researchers in the field became increasingly cognizant of the many variables which were indices of hemispheric dominance and they became increasingly cognizant of the dynamic maturational factors at play in the development of these indices.

One group attempted to ascertain the visual relationships to cortical hemispheric dominance.[32, 33, 34, 35, 36]

[24]Meyers, R. C.: Corpus Callosum and Interhemispheric Communication; Enduring Memory Effects, *Fed. Proc.*, 16:298, 1957.

[25]Meyers, R. C.: Interocular Transfer of Pattern Discrimination in Cats Following Section of Crossed Optic Fibers, *Journ. Comp. and Physiol. Psychol.*, 48:470-473, 1955.

[26]Meyers, R. C.: Function of Corpus Callosum in Interocular Transfer, *Brain*, 79:358-363, 1956.

[27]Stamm, J. S. and Sperry, R. W.: Function of Corpus Callosum in Contralateral Transfer and Somesthetic Discrimination in Cats, *Journ. Comp. and Physiol. Psychol.*, 50:138-143, 1957.

[28]Bremer, F.: La Synergie Interhemispheric, *Strasbourg Med.*, 7:533-552, 1956.

[29]Akelatis, A. J.: Studies on the Corpus Callosum II, The Higher Visual Functions in Each Homonymous Field Following Complete Section of the Corpus Callosum, *Arch. of Neur. and Psychiat.*, 45:788-796, 1941.

[30]Akelatis, A. J.: Studies on the Corpus Callosum, VII, Study of Language Function (tactile and visual lexia and graphia) unilaterally following section of the Corpus Callosum, *Journ. of Neuropath. and Neurol.*, 2:226-262, 1943.

[31]Akelatis, A. J.: A Study of Gnosis, Praxia and Language Following Section of Corpus Callosum and Anterior Commissure, *Journ. of Neursurg.*, I:99-102, 1944.

[32]Scheidman, G.: A Simple Test For Ocular Dominance, *Amer. Journ. of Psychol.*, 43, 1931.

[33]Gates, A. I., and Bond., G. C.: The Relationship of Handedness, Eye Sighting and Acuity Dominance to Reading, *Journ. Ed. Psychol.*, 27:3, 1936.

⟹

This group felt that there might be other clinical indices of hemispheric dominance and they attempted to correlate these indices. This was especially true with the hand-eye correlation.

With advancing knowledge in the field of neurosurgery new techniques were developed which gave us greater insights into cortical functions. Such dramatic surgical procedures as the removal of a hemisphere gave us new physiological and new clinical knowledge of the relationship of language to cortical function.[37, 38, 39]

With greater sophistication of data a natural question arose. The question related to the possibility of ascertaining the dominant cortical hemisphere in a way other than through clinical observations. Wada and co-workers have attempted to develop a procedure for the physiological and biological determination of the dominant cortical hemisphere via the injection of sodium amytal into the intracarotid artery.[40, 41]

This has been followed and reported upon by other workers.[42, 43, 44]

[34]Walls, G. L.: Theory of Ocular Dominance, *Arch. Ophth.*, 45:387, 1951.

[35]Fink., W. H.: The Dominant Eye: Its Clinical Significance, *Arch. Ophth.*, 19:555, April, 1938.

[36]Dearborn, O. W. F.: Ocular and Manual Dominance in Dyslexia, *Psychol. Bull.*, 28:704, 1938.

[37]Krynauw, R. A.: Infantile Hemiplegia Treated by Removing One Cerebral Hemisphere, *Journ. Neurol. Psychiat., Chicago*, 34:234-267, 1935.

[38]Zollinger, R.: Removal of the Left Cerebral Hemisphere, Report of a case, *Arch. Neurol. Psychiat., Chicago*, 34:1005-1064, 1935.

[39]Carmichael, E. A.: Hemispherectomy and The Localization of Function, *Lectures on the Scientific Basis of Medicine*, 3:93-103, 1954.

[40]Wada, J.: A New Method For The Determination of the Side of Cerebral Speech Dominance. A Preliminary Report on the Intra-carotid injection of sodium amytal in man, *Med. Biol.*, 14:221-222, 1949.

[41]Wada J., and Rasmussen, T.: Intra-carotid Injection of Sodium Amytal For the Lateralization of Cerebral Speech Dominance, *Journ. Neurosurg.*, 17:266-282, 1960.

[42]Alema, G. and Donini, G.: Sulle Modificazioni Cliniche ed Elettroen Cefalografiche da Introduzione Intracarotidea di iso-amil-etil- barbiturato di Sodio Nell'uomo, *Bull. Soc. Ital. Sper.*, 36:900-904, 1960.

[43]Terzian, H., and Cecotto, D.: Su Un Nuovo Metodo Per La Determinazione E LoStudio Della Dominanza Emisferico, *Gior. Psichiat. e Neuropat.*, 57:1-35, 1959.

[44]Perria, L., Rosadini, G. and Rossi, F.: Determination of Side of Cerebral Dominance with Amobarbital, *Arch. of Neurol.*, 4:173-181, Feb., 1961.

These researchers have found that speech disturbances coupled with depressed emotional reactions indicate that the dominant hemisphere has been injected by the drug and that no speech disturbance coupled with a euphoric type emotional reaction indicate that the sub-dominant hemisphere has received the drug.

New insights led other researchers to investigate a great number of possible factors relating cortical function to language and behavior. These studies were very varied and there were many of them. The author has chosen to refer to a few representative studies.[45, 46, 47]

The trend was away from the mere correlation of handedness to speech and the approach became more wholistic in nature. Some workers began to investigate birth trauma to the nervous system as an etiological factor in speech and reading retardation.[48, 49]

Eames studied one hundred children with reading difficulties. He separated them into groups; one which was composed of children who were premature at birth and the other full term. He found that the premature group presented more neurological lesions, visual problems, slow recognition speed and lateral variations.[50]

The maturational lag of the nervous system was investigated as a part of the etiological investigations pursued.[51]

Cohn demonstrated with 46 children that delayed communica-

---

[45]Anderson, A. L.: The Effect of Laterality Localization of Focal Brain Lesions on Wechsler-Bellevue Subtests, *Journ. Clin. Psychol.* 7:149-153, 1951.

[46]Smith, K. V.: The Role of the Commissural Systems of the Cerebral Cortex in the Determination of Handedness, Eyedness and Footedness in Man, *Journ. of Gen. Psychol.*, 32:39-79, 1945.

[47]Jervis, G. A., and others: Revascularization of the Brain in Mental Defectives, *Neurology*, 3:871-878, Dec., 1953.

[48]Kawi, A. A., and Pasamanick, B.: Association of Factors of Pregnancy with Reading Disorders in Children, *J. A. M. A., 166*:1420-1423, 1958.

[49]Walker, J.: Foetal Anoxia, *Journ. of Obs. and Gyn. of Br. Emp., 61*:162-180, April, 1954.

[50]Eames, T. H.: Comparison of Children of Premature and Full Term Birth Who Fail in Reading, *Journ. of Ed. Res.*, 38:506-508, March, 1945.

[51]Bender, L.: Specific Reading Disability As A Maturational Lag, *Bull. of Orton Soc.*, 7:9-18, 1951.

tion was primarily an expression of general disturbance or lack of maturation of neurological function as compared with his control group.[52]

Gellner's work indicates a close relationship of neurological dysfunction with the group generally classified as mentally retarded.[53]

This new trend in the research gradually evolved in attempts to deal not only with the details of physiology of the nervous system but some investigators began to deal with the nervous system conceptually and began to relate the whole of the nervous system to behavior. One of the great sources of materials and inspiration came from the work of Lashley. His voluminous work with animals and his brilliant insights into the functional relationships within the central nervous system gave us new and important data relating cortical function to intelligence and language.[54, 55]

Sherrington's pioneering work in the field of neurology and his writings which are the classics in the field helped toward greater understanding and wider acceptance of the relationships of the human nervous system to human behavior.[56, 57, 58]

Burr also dealt with the nervous system as a whole and arrived at conceptual conclusions. He related the basal ganglia to phylogenetically conditioned control of behavior, the brain stem to automatic regulation of chemical factors of the body and the spinal cord to reflex management.[59]

---

[52]Cohn, R.: Delayed Acquisition of Reading and Writing Abilities in Children, *Arch. of Neurol., 4:*153-164, Feb., 1961.

[53]Gellner, L.: *A Neurophysiological Concept of Mental Retardation and Its Educational Implications,* Chicago, Levensen Research Foundation, Cook County Hospital, pp. 1-44, 1959.

[54]Lashley, K. S.: *Brain Mechanisms and Intelligence: a Quantitative Study of Injuries to the Brain,* Chicago, University of Chicago Press, 1929.

[55]Lashley, K. S.: *The Problem of Serial Order in Behavior,* The Hixon Symposium, (L. A. Jefress, Ed.), New York, John Wiley Sons, 1951, pp. 112-135.

[56]Sherrington, C. S.: *The Brain and Its Mechanisms,* London, Oxford University Press, 1933.

[57]Sherrington, C. S.: *Integrative Action of the Nervous System,* New. Ed., Cambridge, Cambridge Univ. Press, 1947.

[58]Sherrington, C. S.: *Man and His Nature,* Cambridge, Cambridge Univ. Press, 1951.

⟫⟫→

The brilliant work of Hebb has become a classic in the explanation of the relationships of various neural levels to the many variables of human behavior, perception and expression. He presents the most plausible neurological explanation of the process of learning to date.[60]

Weiner's work has helped us to understand the function of the brain from a mechanical and feed-back point of view. His views on stuttering are classic in that they bring into full play all of the known knowledge of neurology and explain very plausibly a problem which has baffled us for centuries.[61]

Penfield has pioneered in the localization of cortical function. His rationale for the relationships of cortical function with subcortical functions and their relationships to behavior are modern classics in the field. His voluminous research forms the basis for many modern neurosurgical procedures and modern neurological concepts.[62, 63]

The author has been privileged to work personally with Temple Fay, who gave to the field its first real insight into the relationship of the phylogeny and the ontogeny of human movement. As a result of Fay's monumental work, we can deduce certain phylogenetic-ontogenetic relationships of the entire nervous system.[64, 65]

Spitz, friend and co-worker, has pioneered in the development of the ventriculo-jugular shunt procedure for use in hydrocephalus and has also pioneered in the area of childhood hemispherectomy. These procedures have given us new opportunities to view cortical and sub-cortical functions and to better understand their relationships to both language and mobility functions.[66, 67]

[59]Burr, H. S.: *The Neural Basis of Human Behavior,* Springfield, Thomas, 1960, pp. 1-272.

[60]Hebb, D. O.: *The Organization of Behavior,* New York, John Wiley & Sons, 1949, pp. 1-319.

[61]Weiner, N.: Cybernetics, *Scientific American,* p. 614, November, 1948.

[62]Penfield, W. and Roberts, L.: *Speech and Brain Mechanisms,* Princeton University Press, 1959, pp. 1-286.

[63]Penfield, W., and Rasmussen, T.: *The Cerebral Cortex of Man,* New York, The MacMillan Co., 1950, pp. 1-235.

[64]Fay, T.: *Origin of Human Movement,* Amer. Journ. of Psychiat., 3:644-652, March, 1955.

[65]Fay, T.: Rehabilitation of Patients with Spastic Paralysis, *Journ. Internat. Coll. of Surgeons,* 22:200-203, August, 1954.

⮕

Doman has pioneered in the field of developmental neurology. His work provides us with the developmental clinical concomitants of neurological levels. He has given to the field areas and procedures of clinical measurements which are highly correlated to neurological function and which have in the past been overlooked. His work has provided reliable and valid clinical indices for the ascertainment of neurological maturity.[68]

As we review the general trends of research in the field, we find that there remains a small group which persists in perpetuating the error of equating handedness alone with cortical hemispheric dominance, and then insists that this represents neurological maturity. It can be easily observed that the bulk of the research which is now being conducted is more sophisticated in nature. We are now looking at the entire nervous system wholistically and we are relating its total function to behavior. We are using many variables to ascertain dominance and, indeed, the search goes on. The clinical variables of dominance are becoming more numerous in the literature and, as a result, our ability to ascertain dominance has become more reliable and more valid.

These men, Gesell, Orton, Skeffington, Getman, Harmon, Wada, Eames, Gellner, Lashley, Sherrington, Burr, Hebb, Weiner, Penfield, Roberts, Fay, Spitz and Doman, although representing different biases, have one thing in common—they are all looking for a central and basic approach to solving the problems of language. They all know that when one has an injury to a specific part of the brain his speech and reading functions are changed. They know that they can ameliorate certain problems of communication through surgical procedures. They also know that certain types of injury result in certain types of language problems. In short, the basis of speech and reading is the brain, hence, the treatment of problems of reading and speech should be directed toward the brain.

[66]Spitz, E. B.: Subdural Suppuration Originating in Purulent Leptomeningitis, *Arch. Neurol. and Psychiat.*, 22:144-149, Feb. 1945.

[67]Spitz, E. B., Ziff, M., Brenner, C., Dawson, C.: New Absorbable Material For Use In Neurologic and General Surgery, *Science, 102*:621-622, December, 1945.

[68]Doman G., Delacato, C. H., and Doman, R.: *The Doman-Delacato Developmental Profile*, Philadelphia, The Rehabilitation Center at Philadelphia, 1962.

These men and their work must certainly be noted by educators. This is especially true for those educators whose bias is peripheral in nature. Those educators who feel that phonetics or educational methodology are the real answer to the diagnosis and treatment of speech and reading problems must, of necessity, be stopped short when the neurosurgeon can, with a non-phonetic, a non-methodological and a non-psychological scalpel, significantly change the language function of a human being.

The author must say here that, without the help of these men, this rationale would have been impossible and that, without their work, education would have remained stagnated at the level to which Orton's followers had taken them. Without these men education would still be treating neurological problems by teaching phonetics and we would still be achieving the poor results of the past.

Chapter 4

THE PHYLOGENY OF NEUROLOGICAL
ORGANIZATION

Speech and reading are the most uniquely human activities of man. They precede, are part of, and follow the mysterious yet magnificent human process which we call "ideation."

Only a century ago Darwin published the first scientific insight into the origins of man. That century has been punctuated by many Darwinian debates.

The debates have subsided and modern scientific opinion is typified by the following:

"At last week's Chicago meeting of the American Association for the Advancement of Science, Harvard's George Gaylord Simpson, Vertebrate paleontologist, seized upon the centenary of Darwin's publication of the Origin of Species to summarize today's consensus of scientific thinking on the nature and origin of man. The ancestry of man is still not fully known, he conceded, but he denounced "pussyfooting" about apes in man's family tree.

"Apologists emphasize that man cannot be a descendant of any living ape, and go on to state that man is not really descended from an ape or monkey at all but from an earlier common ancestor. In fact that common ancestor would certainly be called an ape or monkey in popular speech by anyone who saw it. Since the terms 'ape' and 'monkey' are defined by popular usage, man's ancestors were apes or monkeys (or successively both) . . . Man is in the fullest sense a part of nature and not apart from it. He is not figuratively but literally akin to every living thing, be it an amoeba, a tapeworm, a flea, a seaweed, an oak tree or a monkey." In a word, man lives in a world "in which he is not the darling of the gods."

[26]

In other species, Simpson points out, uncontrolled evolution often leads to degeneration and usually to extinction. "But man is not just another animal. He is unique in peculiar and extraordinarily significant ways. He is the only organism with true language. This makes him the only animal who can store knowledge and pass it on beyond individual memory." . . .[1]

To be totally human man must be able to use language. Language in man is the result of the phylogenetic development of the nervous system. Language in the development of an individual is the result of the development and organization of his nervous system. Man differs in this development from primates and lower forms of animals in that he has added the final lateral progression to this phylogenetic development. Individuals who have normal language development have achieved this uniquely human final lateral progression. Those who have difficulty with language in the form of speaking or reading have not achieved this final lateral progression or in some cases have not completed the vertical progression.

Plant and animal life could not help but change during the last half billion years. They changed in many ways in adapting to a dramatically changing and unpredictable environment.

Let us scan the past half billion years for some environmental variations which could not help but have significant effects on the origins of human movement and human communication.

CLIMATE

Cambrian

The climate of the Cambrian period was probably mild with climatic belts less sharply defined than at present. Deposits of pure limestone even at high latitudes attest to this.

Ordovician

The climate of this period was much warmer than at present with mild conditions extending into the Arctic. Climatic zones were poorly marked.

---

[1] *Time Magazine,* Science Section, January 11, 1960.

Silurian

After a probable slight cooling in the early Silurian, mild temperatures again extended into the Arctic during the middle Silurian as indicated by the wide extent of limestones and dolomites. In late Silurian time arid conditions were prevalent and long periods of drought were caused by the flatness of the continents.

Devonian

A mild climate with a lack of strongly marked climatic belts continued, but the upland slopes of rising mountains were more humid than the basins and lowlands.

Mississippian

The climate of the Mississippian period was apparently very changeable with humidity over the lands differing from region to region and from time to time. A warm climate is indicated for most of the period by the abundance of crinoids, but in Australia there is evidence that glaciation took place although its exact date is not certain.

Pennsylvanian

A warm persistently moist climate prevailed over most of the earth. Coral reefs and insects of very large size indicate tropical conditions even in the Arctic. It was a period of lofty mountains with only local aridity.

Permian

A withdrawal of the sea and lofty mountains caused local extremes of climates. Deserts were probably widespread and arid conditions prevailed over most of the world. There was a brief epoch of ice ages in the early Permian.

Triassic

An arid or semi-arid climate was remarkably widespread, and moderately warm temperatures extended into the Arctic.

Jurassic

The Jurassic was more humid than the Triassic and more mild than at present. Insects were large and dinosaurs roamed as far north as Alberta and Mongolia, both facts indicating a warm climate.

Cretaceous

The early Cretaceous was considerably cooler than the previous period and some ice caps were developed. In late Cretaceous time, however, the seas spread and the climate became mild over most of the earth. A second drop in temperature occurred at the end of this period.

Tertiary

The climate was milder, more humid and more uniform during the Paleocene, Eocene and Oligocene than at the present time. In the Oligocene, however, there was a gradual cooling that became more marked in the Pliocene and culminated in the Pleistocene with the Ice Ages. Rising mountains in the latter part of the Tertiary made the climate more diversified.[2]

Pleistocene

Four major advances of glaciation took place in this short (3,000,000 years) division of geologic time with ice sheets reaching into moderate latitudes of Europe and North America. The last advance took place 10,700 years ago after which the ice melted and retreated in a few thousand years. During the three prolonged interglacial periods the climate was sometimes even milder than at present though never reaching the level of the preceding 100,000,000 years. The mean temperature during the Pleistocene varied between 36° F and 62° F whereas the present temperature is 58° F and throughout most of geologic history it was 72° F.

Recent

Evidence of fossil plants and of other lines established beyond doubt that the climate reached a maximum of warmth and dryness between 6000 and 4000 years ago. Since then, with minor fluctuations, it has become cooler and more moist down to the middle of the last century when glaciers reached a maximum.

---

[2]Dunbar, Carl O.: *Historical Geology*, New York, John Wiley and Sons, Inc., 1949.

During the last one hundred years or so a warming trend has occurred with glaciers shrinking at a very rapid rate.[3]

TEMPERATURE

Geological and paleontological studies give us some indication of ancient temperatures but at best the results are approximations and exceedingly incomplete considering the long period of geological history. A new tool, however, has recently been discovered by means of which temperatures have been dated more accurately back to 80,000,000 years ago or to the Cretaceous period. This method involves a study of isotopes of oxygen in marine fossils and sediments.

One of the interesting outcomes of this research is the discovery that all the glacial periods occurred in only 3,000,000 years and that, therefore, the evolution of man and mammals occurred during this time, at a much greater rate than hitherto thought. Another result is the discovery of fluctuations in temperature 65,000,000 years ago that probably brought about the extinction of dinosaurs and other animals.[4]

OXYGEN

During the Precambrian and early part of the Paleozoic periods oxygen was formed by the photochemical decomposition of water vapor, but was used in combination with carbon monoxide to form carbon dioxide. There was, therefore, little free oxygen in the earth's atmosphere until plant life developed on land in the Silurian and photosynthesis greatly increased the oxygen production rate. Presumably the amount of oxygen in the atmosphere increased rapidly as vegetation spread over the continents and then reached an equilibrium which has probably been offset one way or the other by the relative amount of vegetation on earth. Thus, a drought or an ice age may conceivably have affected the amount of oxygen in the air.[5]

[3]Flint, Richard F.: *Glacial Geology and the Pleistocene Epoch,* New York, John Wiley and Sons, Inc., Second Printing, January, 1948.

[4]Emiliani, Cesare: Ancient Temperatures, *Scientific American,* February, 1958.

[5]Dunbar, Carl O.: *Historical Geology,* New York, John Wiley and Sons, Inc., 1949, page 201.

OZONE

Ozone is formed from oxygen by ultraviolet rays in the stratosphere. Therefore, as the amount of oxygen increased in the Silurian, so did, presumably, the amount of ozone and this, in turn, resulted in effective shielding of ultraviolet radiations dangerous to cells. There is only the merest trace of ozone at ground level and this is carried down by wind currents from the stratosphere. As a result, there is a seasonal and daily variation in the amount of ozone at ground level. A variation with latitude has also been observed, there being less ozone near the equator. Variations in the ozone level in the stratosphere, and these could have been profound though unknown in the geologic past, may have had considerable effect on life on earth through ineffective shielding.[6, 7]

NITROGEN

Atmospheric nitrogen unites with oxygen and other elements to form simple chemicals such as nitrates which are dissolved by rain water and absorbed by plants. Nitrogen then undergoes a complicated cycle through the biosphere with a turnover period of about one hundred million years. Hence, the abundance of plant and animal life would affect the nitrogen equilibrium to some extent, and it would appear that, when life on earth was on the increase, nitrogen would be taken from the atmosphere and, when on the decrease, it would be given back through decay. Because nitrogen forms a major portion of the atmosphere any variations in the geologic past would have been relatively small.

CARBON DIOXIDE

The earth's atmosphere received its carbon dioxide chiefly from volcanic sources and for some billions of years was probably considerably more plentiful than after the Silurian period. At that time plant life spread over the earth and carbon was extracted from CO_2 and oxygen given up to the atmosphere.

---

[6]Bates, D. R., (Ed.): *The Earth and Its Atmosphere*, New York, Basic Books, Inc., 1957.
[7]Cook, S. Gordon: *Our Astonishing Atmosphere*, New York, The Dial Press, 1957.

CO_2 in the earth's present atmosphere constitutes some .03 per cent of its total mass, but this amount can vary widely according to the degree of photosynthesis, the amount of erosion occurring on the continents and according to the temperature of the atmosphere and oceans. The last has a pronounced effect and it is known that when the temperature of the earth is lower, the amount of CO_2 is less. But whether a decrease in CO_2 in the atmosphere causes a lowering in temperature or whether a lowering in temperature brings on a decrease in CO_2 is not definitely known, although the former is suspected. At any rate, it is known that for the past several hundred million years most of the world has had a tropical climate with considerably more CO_2 in the atmosphere. Every 250 million years or so, however, as in the Permian period, and during the last half million years, there have been relatively short glacial periods when the world temperature was considerably cooler and the amount of CO_2 in the atmosphere as much as 50 per cent less. Thus, at present, there is less CO_2 in the atmosphere than throughout much of geologic history but somewhat more than at the height of each of four glacial maxima during the recent glacial epoch. The fractional volume abundance of CO_2 rose by 9 per cent between 1900 and 1935 as a result of industrial fuel consumption and of the change in the ratio of agricultural to forest land. In 1000 years, it is thought that we will have increased the concentration of CO_2 ten times and the earths temperature at or near ground level will be 22 degrees warmer. The temperature will then begin to fall as CO_2 is taken up by the oceans.[8, 9]

ARGON

Most argon isotope A^{40} in the terrestrial atmosphere (as opposed to original or cosmic argon A^{36} of which there is only a trace) was formed by the decay of radioactive potassium isotope K^{40} during the period of earth melting which occurred about five billion years ago. There were also subsequent additions resulting

---

[8]Plass, Gilbert N.: Carbon Dioxide and Climate, *Scientific American*, July, 1959.
[9]For a possible use of Carbon Dioxide as a therapeutic Modality in dealing with brain injured children who have language problems see: Delacato, C., The Treatment and Prevention of Reading Problems, Springfield, Thomas, 1959.

from partial remelting of the earth's crust from time to time. Thus the increase of argon A^{40} since the Cambrian period or the last tenth of earth time must have been slight but somewhat accelerated during periods of widespread erosion.

CARBON MONOXIDE

Before there was plant life on earth and, therefore, before there was abundant oxygen, carbon monoxide, originating from volcanoes, must have been an important constituent of the atmosphere. With an increase in the amount of oxygen, however, in the Silurian period, carbon monoxide was converted to carbon dioxide and there remained only a trace of the former. Soil micro-organisms also played an important part in destroying carbon monoxide.

METHANE

Methane is produced by decaying vegetation in marshes and soil and from natural fuel beds. The amount in the atmosphere is thought to be in equilibrium and to remain nearly constant, although it probably changes slightly with variations in the amount and kind of vegetation on earth. There would presumably have been more methane when the continents were warm and humid and less when drought or glacial conditions prevailed.

HYDROGEN

Hydrogen is formed in the atmosphere when water vapor is decomposed by solar ultraviolet light. It is lost to space, however, about as fast as it is formed because its atoms are so light they reach the escape velocity in the high temperatures of the upper atmosphere. There has probably never been more than a trace of hydrogen in the earth's atmosphere.

HELIUM

Helium is a very rare constituent in the earth's atmosphere and is made up of isotope mass 4 units and isotope mass 3 units. The latter is present in one millionth the amount of the former, and its source may be extra-terrestrial. The former is formed by the disintegration of radioactive substances in the crust and also as a product of natural springs and natural gas deposits. Like hydrogen, helium escapes the gravitational attraction of the earth and could never have been present in an appreciable amount. During periods of mountain building and rapid erosion there may have been an increase in the liberation of helium through radioactive decay and, therefore, a slight, though probably negligible, increment in its amount in the atmosphere.

NITROUS OXIDE

The trace of nitrous oxide in the atmosphere owes its origin to either certain chemical reactions in the lower atmosphere or to the work of micro-organisms in the soil. Thus, if the latter is valid, when the continents were warm and humid, there could have been an increase in the nitrous oxide production. Even so the amount of nitrous oxide in the atmosphere could never have been significant because it is rapidly destroyed by sunlight.[10]

VOLCANIC DUST

Volcanic dust, as opposed to other atmospheric dust, the amount of which probably varies with changing climates, is present in the atmosphere in direct proportion to the amount of volcanic activity. There have been several periods of increased volcanism since the Cambrian as in the Tertiary, Triassic, Devonian and Ordovician, and during these periods the supply of sunlight must have been temporarily restricted, bringing about changes in climate and lowering of temperatures. These, in turn, would affect several other elements of the earth's environment including life itself.

RADIOACTIVITY

Radioactivity decay in the upper mantle and in the earth's crust has diminished at a nearly constant rate since the beginning of geological time. However, the reduction in the amount of radioactivity since the Cambrian; that is, in the last one-tenth

---

[10]Bates, D. R., (Ed.): *The Earth and Its Atmosphere*, New York, Basic Books, Inc., 1957.

of geologic time must have been slight. Radioactivity at ground level may be somewhat increased when the continents are high and broad and the processes of erosion operating at a maximum. Variation in the intensity of radioactivity from space would be difficult to evaluate but would presumably be chiefly related to solar fluctuations.

Some chemicals (so-called radiomimetic chemicals) have the same effect on animal cells as do high energy radioactive radiations and are thought to act directly on the genetic material DNA. Some are: epoxies, ethylene imines, esters of methane, sulfonic acid, mustard gas, nitrogen mustard and chlorambucil.[11]

SOLAR RADIATION AND COSMIC RAYS

Since its birth six billion years ago the sun has increased its diameter and its brightness very slowly and has now reached the point where its brightness is 20 to 25 per cent greater than it was initially. Thus, since the Cambrian period the increase in brightness would be about one-tenth of this or 2 or 2½ per cent. But because the total amount of radiation increases more quickly than does the brightness, it may be guessed that the former has increased perhaps 10 or more per cent since the Cambrian. Fluctuations in solar radiation amounting to 3 percent of its average value is a recorded fact and, of course, larger variations may have occurred in the past. A general increase in radiation through geologic time would not only increase the temperature of the world (through infra red), but brings added amounts of x-rays and ultraviolet. Fortunately, a large percentage of these radiations is absorbed in the atmosphere, but a change in the amounts that do reach the earth's surface could have an effect on life because x-rays produce mutations in genes and ultraviolet light destroys cells. The nature of the atmosphere, then (see ozone), along with an increase in solar radiation and of fluctuations in solar radiation determines the amount of radiation that reaches ground level.

---

[11]Alexander, Peter: Radiation—Imitation Chemicals, *Scientific American*, July, 1959.

The very impact of these great environmental variations could not help but be reflected in changes in both plant and animal life.

Let us view man phylogenetically. He is the result of specialization of function beginning with the early vertebrates.

Neurologically up to the level of the vertebrate there was little specialization of function. Prior to the vertebrate in the *phylogenetic* scale the most complex brain was that of the insect. It consisted simply of two ganglia.

For our purposes let us analyze the lowest level of living vertebrates the sharks (dog fish), rays and chimaevas of the Class Chandrichthyes.

They are the earliest form of vertebrates which have complete and separate vertebrae, movable jaws and paired appendages. These vertebrates all live in water. They move by laterally undulating the spine or by vertically undulating the pectoral fins. Both these motions are controlled through the spinal cord.

Anatomically the brain of this class contains rudimentary higher areas but both in size and dominance of function the Medulla is the most important neural area (see Fig. 2).

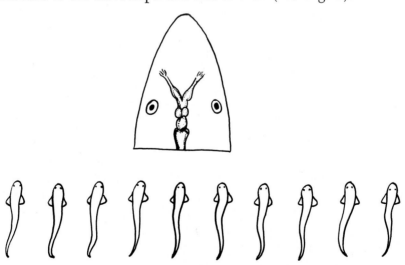

Figure 2. The undulating mobility function of the fish is controlled by the medulla and spinal cord. Note that these areas predominate in the structure of the nervous system of the fish.

The next higher class of vertebrates are the amphibians. Amphibians spend part of their lives in water and part on land. Examples of this class are salamanders and frogs.

The transition from water to land entailed many changes for the amphibian. The amphibian needed sense organs that functioned both in water and on land, changes in circulation to provide for respiration of air, development of lungs, and the amphibian developed limbs instead of fins.

Neurologically the amphibian developed a larger pons and a more dominant mid-brain. These two ganglia vacillated in dominance as the environment required.

While in water the amphibian moves in a homo-lateral pattern as dictated by the pons.

The Salamander in water moves by homolateral strokes of the appendages on one side of the body; alternating body sides, i.e., first he pushes with both limbs on the right side going in the same direction, then with both limbs on the left side going in

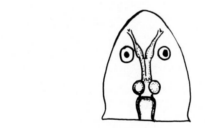

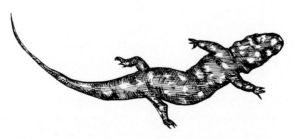

Figure 3. The salamander moves in a homolateral pattern while in water. The Pons becomes the predominant physiological structure of the nervous system where mobility is homolateral. Compare this mobility synergy with sleep patterns in Figures 7 and 8.

the same direction. This is also true for the tadpole when he first develops limbs (see Fig. 3).

When on land, however, the amphibian becomes the first animal which raises its trunk off the ground. Its movement pattern changes dramatically at this point, and it moves in a cross-pattern, i.e., its fore-limb on the right and the hind limb on the left are pushed at the same time, then alternating to the fore-limb on the left and the hind limb on the right (see Fig. 4).

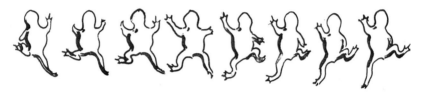

Figure 4. The amphibian, when on *land*, moves in a cross-pattern. Note the beginning of the use of opposite limbs in this mobility synergy. As the *right* fore-limb moves forward the *left* hind-limb moves forward. The synergy ends in the opposite phase with the *left* fore-limb forward and the *right* hind-limb forward.

The amphibian has transitioned from a water to land animal, from a homo-lateral to a cross-pattern animal and from a pons to a mid-brain animal.

The amphibian brain looks like an expanded end to the spinal cord. Going from the cord anteriorly we first find the Medulla, which gives rise to most of the cranial nerves. Running in a thin transverse line over the Medulla is the Cerebellum. Anteriorly we see the optic lobes, which serve to inhibit spinal cord reflexes rather than deal primarily with vision, and anterior to it we have the epiphysis and the pituitary. The anterior brain contains the olfactory lobes, part of which make up the cerebral hemispheres. These can be removed surgically and the animal continues to respond in almost normal fashion to stimulation.

If we surgically remove the anterior portion of the brain of a frog and place him in water, he swims in a normal fashion. If we surgically remove the anterior portion of the brain of the salamander (so that we interfere with some area of the mid-brain) he swims in the normal fashion (homolaterally) but when placed on land can no longer walk in the normal cross-pattern. He reverts to homolateral attempts at movement on land and cannot move with his belly off the ground. He loses the third dimension.

The next higher class of development is the reptile. This class includes lizards, turtles, crocodiles and alligators. The young reptile need not be immersed in water at any time during his life so that the reptile class is the first true land animal that has evolved. Their circulatory system is much more complex than that of the amphibian class. They have a nearly completely divided ventricle in the heart, resulting in a four-chambered heart much like that of the mammal. They have a nearly complete diaphragm separating the chest and abdominal cavities.

Anatomically, reptiles have a comparatively large mid-brain. This is the most significant neural development over the amphibian stage. The reptile always moves in a cross-pattern (see Fig. 5).

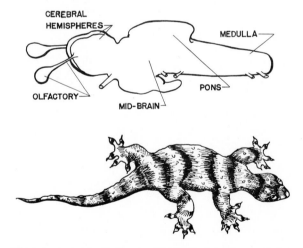

Figure 5. The movement of the reptile is truly cross-pattern. Note that the opposite extremities furnish the propulsive movement simultaneously. The *left* fore-limb and the *right* hind-limb propel and then the *right* fore-limb and the *left* hind-limb propel. Also note the increased size of the mid-brain as related to the other portions of the reptilian central nervous system.

The next higher class is mammals. This class has an increase in the size of the cortex (see Fig. 6).

The phylogenetic level nearest to the level of man is the primate level.

Primates are mammals. They usually have five digits on their hands and have flat nails instead of claws. They have prehensile hands and feet instead of opposing digits. Their brains contain

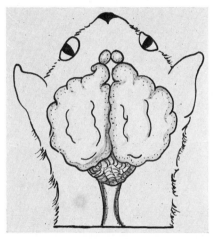

Figure 6. The mammal's brain is typified by a dramatic increase in the size of the cortex. Compare the relative size of the cat's cortex with that of the reptilian cortex in Figure 5.

a cortex which is most similar to the cortex of man. In higher forms cortical convolutions are present.

Primates are divided into three groups:

1. **Lemuroids**

    They are the least highly evolved of the primates. They have unwrinkled and unexpressive faces with eyes set in the sides of the head. Their visual fields overlap very little and the retina lacks both a fovea and a macula. As a result, they have no stereopsis. The face is expressionless, the only expression coming from jerky movements of the eyes, eye lids and ears.

2. **Tarsoidea**

    He is more erect and moves by hopping. His forebrain is broader and he has a differentiated visual area in the brain. His back legs are used for support and his fore legs are used for prehension. He feeds himself with his hands (bi-manually) and he uses his facial muscles for expression. His eyes are set more forward in his head, hence his visual fields are more overlapping but he has no stereopsis.

3. Anthropoidea

This group includes monkeys and anthropoid apes. They have a larger fore-brain, a more convoluted cortex and occipital lobes which overhang the mid-brain. Their eyes are frontally directed, and they begin to have stereoscopic vision. They are adaptable for an upright position. They begin crawling from five to seven months of age, and during the second half of the first year they begin to walk both quadrupedly (creeping) and bipedly. Their communication relies on postures, gestures, physical contact and thudding.

This group shows some preference for a particular hand, foot or eye but definite right-sidedness or definite left-sidedness has not been established for any anthropoid type.[12]

Up to this point in the phylogenetic process we note that two basic human factors are missing; language and sidedness or laterality. The primates develop bilateral and binocular functions. They never develop single handedness and they have never had language. We must move on to early man to see the first indications of both handedness and language.

It is well known that Americans, Europeans and undoubtedly all civilized people of the world are predominantly right handed. It is possible, though, that predominant right handedness is a product of the activities of civilization such as handicraft, eating, writing, sports and military service, etc. With this question in mind, we examined photographs of aborigines engaged in using an arm for one purpose or another and were able to determine their handedness. The results of this investigation are tabulated as follows:

---

[12]Hooten: *Why Men Behave Like Apes and Vice-Versa,* Princeton University Press, 1941.

Aborigines	Photos Right Hand Users	Photos Left Hand Users
Canadian and N. Greenland Eskimos	43	3
Maori	5	0
Natives of Borneo	17	0
Natives of Luzon (1911)	18	1
Central African Tribes	8	2
Easter Islanders	2	0
Indians of British Guiana	15	0
	108	6

It is apparent from these limited observations that present day aborigines throughout the world are also right handed and that therefore predominant right handedness is universal and not necessarily a function of civilization.

An apparently anomalous situation exists, however, in southern Iraq where the prevailing culture requires that individuals use one arm for certain definite activities and the other for certain other activities—they have a so-called "clean" and "dirty" hand. As a result, a very high level of ambidexterity has been achieved among these people, and they could mistakenly be considered left handed.[13]

Having established that all present peoples are predominantly right handed, we decided to look back in history to the time of the ancient Greeks and Romans. Here again predominant right handedness was proved by an examination of the art of the time. Sculptors' models held the discus, shot the bow, or balanced the javelin with their right hands. Further evidence is given by a classical archaeologist who states that "the word sinister (left) had already come to mean awkward in the classical period," and that "soldiers carried their shields on their left arms and their spears in their right hands, and statesmen could not have gestured with their left arm when their togas were properly draped."[14]

Looking farther back in time, back to the most recent ice age, 18,000 B.C., we find still further evidence that man, even in that remote time, was mainly right handed. This suggests that the cave dwellers were mainly right handed. This suggestion is

---

[13]Garvin, Maxwell: *People of the Reeds*, New York, Harper & Co., 1957.
[14]Blake, M. E.: Fellow American Academy in Rome, Personal Communication, 1961.

strongly supported by a study of handprints found in many caves where, in the majority of examples, the left hand was placed against the wall and its outline traced in paint with the right hand, thus indicated right handedness. It should be noted that these right handed Aurignacian stone age people were a part of the already diversified Cromagnon species which was the ancestor of all races living today.[15]

Another line of research which involves a study of ancient skulls was followed by G. Elliot Smith who, in 1927, found that in right handed persons the sulcus lunatus in the visual area of the brain is on the left side, and that in left handed persons it is on the right side. Further study by Elliot Smith revealed the existence of a ridge (crista Lunata) in the endocranial aspect of the skull that corresponds to the sulcus lunatus. He was thus able to conclude that certain individual skulls of ancient man were possessed by either left or right handed people. According to him the "Lady of Lloyds" (upper Paleolithic) and the original Pithecanthropus were left handed and the "LaChapelle" man and Eoanthropus were right handed. In the Rhodesian man, however, the lunate cristae were symmetrical as in the Anthropoid apes, which indicates ambidexterity.

These studies were apparently made on a few skulls and cannot indicate the actual predominant handedness in any of the mentioned human types. However, a study of ancient skulls and of humeri and clavicles which, according to Wood-Jones, also show variation with handedness and footedness may well lead to concrete results that could be compared with evidence from other sources.[16]

Australopithecus (prometheus), a proto-human unearthed in South Africa from deposits thought to be nearly 1,000,000 years old, has for some time been considered a missing link between the anthropoid and man. This "ape-man" or "man-ape" stood erect, fashioned weapons from bone and represented a culture that predated the old stone age. His chief weapon was the arm

[15]Bibby, Geoffrey: *The Testimony of the Spade*, New York, Alfred Knopf, Inc., 1956.

[16]Gates, Reginald R.: *Human Genetics*, New York, The MacMillan Co., 1946, pp. 912-13.

bone of the antelope with which he skillfully bludgeoned the animals of his environment and, if sufficiently hungry, his fellows. The most sought-after animal was the baboon and, in the deposits of this period, its skeletons appear in abundance. An investigation of the baboon skulls by Professor Dart revealed that, of 42 crushed skulls, 40 were crushed on the left side, indicating with little doubt that Australopithecus was right-handed.

The line of evolution that led to Australopithecus and subsequently to true man branched from the anthropoid line of evolution, it is believed, in the Miocene epoch of the Tertiary period, or about 20,000,000 years ago. Apparently righthandedness was developed at some time between 1,000,000 years ago and 20,-000,000 years ago, the anthropoids being ambidextrous.[17]

If right eyedness followed the course of right handedness in evolution, and this does not seem unlikely, specialization on the right side may conceivably have been a critical factor in the rapid development of human intelligence.

Man's great contribution to the process of phylogenetics has not been one of structure, but has been one of function. Man differs from the primates in that he has added a lateral development to his neurological organization. When this lateral development is completed, man becomes a speaking and reading being; if this development is not completed some developmental lag in language occurs.

There is considerable evidence that man achieved the bipedal position and laterality because of his tools. Recently, tools have been found with man-apes indicating that ambidextrous primates used very crude tools. We can hypothesize that the continued use of one handed tools biased early man toward one sidedness for more efficient use of the tools.[18]

If one juxtaposes the result of the use of tools, the development of handedness with the beginning of speech and music, one readily sees that speech appears phylogenetically with handedness. The progress from the primate is (a) tools, (b) using the

[17]Dart, Raymond A. and Craig, Dennis: *Adventures with the Missing Link*, New York, Harper & Bros., 1959, p. 106.

[18]For an excellent treatment of this subject see, Washburn, Sherwood L., Tools and Human Evolution, Scientific American, 203 pp. 63-75, Sept., 1960.

tools with a preferred hand, (c) cortical hemispheric dominance, (d) then speech and music. This chronology is the result of function determining organization as an extension of the premise of function determining structure. Primates have no vowels (color) or music as part of their communication system.[19]

The relationship of the establishment of one sidedness to the development of speech, the relationship of the establishment of one sidedness to music and the subsequent relationship of speech and reading to music are important relationships. The author feels that speech was developed when cortical hemispheric dominance began to become established. The author feels, further, that speech and eventually reading are controlled by the dominant hemisphere which has developed and that at this point in the evolutionary process, when a dominant-sub-dominant hemisphere relationship emerged, speech emerged and was controlled by the dominant hemisphere and music emerged and was controlled by the sub-dominant hemisphere.

"Trauma of the controlling hemisphere results in loss of language skills, but, equally important, trauma of the sub-dominant area results in loss of tonal factors. Left hemiplegics (right handed people who have suffered a cerebrovascular accident to the right, or sub-dominant hemisphere of the cortex) have no difficulty with speech but suffer loss in tonal memory, tonal appreciation and the ability to carry a tune."[20]

"As is well known in dealing with people who have cortical damage, if the cortex on the side of the body which is the sub-dominant side is damaged (dominant cortical hemisphere) we find a condition called aphasia, or the inability to communicate. These people are unable to speak or to read. One of the well known techniques for helping such people to regain functional speech is using tonality. Although these people have damage in what is the dominant hemisphere of the cortex (the skill side) the sub-dominant side remains intact and in this area tonality finds its basis. If one takes such a patient and asks him to sing a

[19]Hockett, C. F.: The Origin of Speech, *Scientific American*, 203, pp. 89-96, Sept., 1960.

[20]Delacato, C. H.: *The Treatment and Prevention of Reading Problems*, Springfield, Thomas, 1959, pp. 21-22.

familiar song, one finds that he can speak all the words of the tune, can sing such songs as Happy Birthday to You and say his own name in it as long as he is singing. When the song is over, he is unable to say his name. The only conclusion we can reach is that the tonality carried the skill section, tonality being in the non-affected area or sub-dominant hemisphere. . . .

"We have heard of the many cases of stuttering which do not stutter when singing. Music teachers have been historically amazed with this phenomenon. The author feels that stuttering is the result of too much hemispheric balance. There is no dominance, hence we have a stutter. If we add tonality, the hemisphere which controls tonality and which is normally the sub-dominant hemisphere becomes dominant and the stutter disappears."[21]

As we assess man, the ultimate product of the phylogenetic process, we find that he retains many of the lower level reactive patterns which preceded him. We find that he differs from the Primates in that he:

1. Stands fully upright.
2. Is able to supinate and pronate his hand and forearm.
3. Has an opposable finger and thumb instead of prehensile grasp.
4. Has functional stereoscopic vision.
5. Has developed lateral dominance.
6. Has developed a symbolic language.

These six factors enable man to rule our planet.

These six factors are the result of adaptive activities necessitated by a changing environment. As the environment changed, man had to change his activity or function. As his function changed, his very structure changed. Hence, his present structure is the result of his past and present function.

If this is true with the phylogenetic development of mankind, is it not possible that ontogenetically we can change the structure of a single man (sic. child) by altering his environment and function?

Now let us for a moment superimpose the phylogenetic neural structure upon man's neural structure. The progression is obvious and the progression is very logical.

[21]Ibid.

Chapter 5

THE ONTOGENY OF NEUROLOGICAL ORGANIZATION

THE BIOGENETIC Law which states that ontogeny recapitulates phylogeny is an accepted generalization. Let us trace the onto-genetic development of a single human being in terms of neuro-logical organization and structure and let us relate them to phylogeny if possible.

The progression of neurological organization proceeds ver-tically to the cortex as myelenization takes place. These progres-sive organizational stages are chronologically predictable. The orderly and sequential myelinization and organization of the sub-cortical areas is prerequisite to the subsequent proper or-ganization at the level of cortex. They are both prerequisite to the establishment of complete hemispheric dominance.

This progression begins during gestation and is normally com-plete by eight years of age. During gestation and up to the time of birth the spinal cord and medulla oblongata are the upper reaches of neurological organization. Here lie the ancient and primitive reflexes whose basic contribution to neurological or-ganization are muscle tone, reflex movement and the preservation of life. The medullary functions continue of primary importance at the time of birth since they reflexly control such vital life preserving functions as cardio-vascular activity, gastro-intestinal activity and breathing reflexes. At this level, mobility is undulat-ing and fish-like in character. As the newborn makes the transi-tion from a fluid to a gaseous environment proper medullary function is vital to survival.

The infant at this level has movement but no mobility. His movements consist of crude trunkal movements not oriented to-ward any objectives. It is a totally reflex synergy.

[47]

All of the infant's activities at this stage are reflex in nature. His visual reactions, his sucking reactions and his crying reactions are all on a purely involuntary level. These reflex activities require relatively short and uncomplicated neural pathways. All of the reactions are of a survival nature.

The infant lives at this level until about sixteen weeks of age, at which time he leaves his fish-like existence and moves on to the next level of neurological organization.

The next higher level is the amphibian-like level which is the responsibility of the pons. The pons lies just above the medulla oblongata. The occulo-motor nuclei extend down through the mid-brain to the floor of the fourth ventricle, which is in the upper portion of the pons. Auditory pathways cross the midline as do the visual pathways. The decussation for the auditory pathways takes place at a lower level than does the decussation for the visual pathways. The auditory pathways decussate in the floor of the fourth ventrical which is located in the upper portion of the pons. We must note here that although both visual and auditory pathways decussate, the crossing over is only partial for there are some fibers which stay on the same side for both hearing and vision. We can see that at the level of pons we have pathway representation for both visual-motor function and for audition. They are the crudest and phylogenetically the oldest such representations.

The pons is the physiological seat of the tonic neck reflex. Ontogenetically this reflex should be partially established prior to birth and its reflex function tends to cease at about twenty weeks of age. The first use of the tonic neck reflex takes place intra-uterinely. The mere turning of the head flexes the arm and leg toward which the head is turned. The tonic neck reflex allows the foetus its higher level of serialized movement. An intact tonic neck reflex pattern is prerequisite to non-traumatic or normal birth. Obstetrical procedures make use of the tonic neck reflex via the rotation of the baby's head during the birth process. If it is not present at birth, the birth process is made much more difficult. Indeed, many neurological dysfunctions which have as their etiology birth trauma, are probably foetuses which, through some mechanism, had been neurologically injured or neurologically under-developed prior to birth. This trauma results in the lack of a strong tonic neck reflex. As a result, the birth process is made more difficult. The neurological trauma is, therefore, not the result of birth trauma but is, instead, the result of faulty pre-birth neurological development.

An intact tonic neck reflex can function most effectively while the infant is lying on its back. While on its back the child can flex or extend either side of its body simply by turning its head. Since we have been placing babies on their stomachs more and more recently, we find that the proper expression of the tonic neck reflex is interfered with by gravity. When one turns an infant over onto its stomach for sleep, one can see that the weight of the arm and leg on the bed and the friction resulting from their weight makes it very difficult for the arm and leg toward which the head is turned to flex and the opposite arm and leg to extend. Hence, by merely placing the child on its stomach or allowing the child to roll over on its stomach without posturalizing the body in the proper tonic neck position, may be causing an interference to neurological organization. Current data indicates that placing children on their stomachs for sleep is desirable. We must, however, preserve the integrity of the tonic neck reflex by placing the limbs in proper posturalization when we have our children sleep on their stomachs.

The tonic neck reflex is used functionally by the infant for propulsion while the body is dragged along.

This is crawling. You will note that the body remains in contact with the floor at this stage of mobility and that the propulsive movements are made in a homolateral fashion typical of the amphibian, (see page 37) that is, with the arm and leg on the same side of the body flexed and the arm and leg on the opposite side of the body extended. Babies begin to crawl very early in life. Watching babies in the newborn nursery one can readily see the very normal and reflex qualities of this very natural form of mobility. One can also easily observe the reflex character of the tonic neck reflex by placing such an infant on his back and turning his head from side to side. The infant's arms and legs will follow the homolateral patterns described above.

This early crawling is the first mobility function where mobility from one point to another is the result. This mobility pattern vanishes when the child moves on to the mid-brain level. It remains vestigially a part of the nervous system, however. It can be observed in older children while they are asleep. Children who are well organized at the level of pons sleep on their stomachs in a homolateral position typical of the level of pons. Left-handed children tend to sleep in one position and right-handed children in another (see Figs. 7 and 8).

The behavior now results in moving from one place to another, both vision and audition become important receptive modalities.

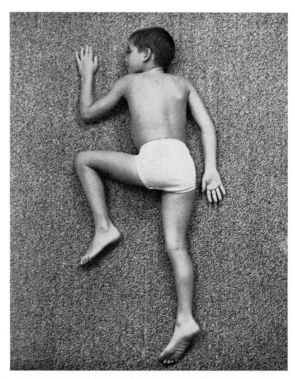

Figure 7. The ideal sleep position of the completely *right*-sided child. This homolateral position is the same as the homolateral position used in early crawling at the level of Pons.

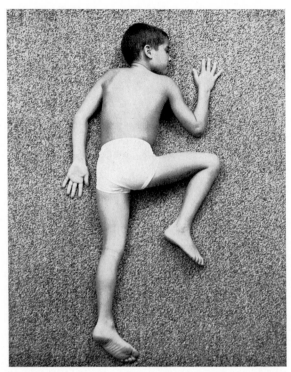

Figure 8. The ideal sleep position of the completely *left*-handed child. This is the opposite phase from Figure 7 as used in proper homolateral crawling. In each of these sleep patterns the thumb on the sub-dominant hand is in the sucking position.

The infant begins to hear himself and to hear the sounds about him. He cannot place them in space but initiates a crude system of conditioned reactions to sound. He uses the ears independent of each other.

Vision at this level is bi-ocular, that is, the eyes are used alternately and rarely in concert. The very position of the eyes in the crawling position precludes their being used in concert, for as one eye is looking, the other is occluded by the floor-cheek contact. As one looks at babies at this level one generally sees a lack of "yoking" of the two eyes. The baby's eyes present a picture of what would be termed later in life, a strabismus. He is unable to use the two eyes in concert. We can see this same phenomenon in the amphibian whose eyes are placed at the sides of his head and whose visual function is also bi-ocular.

We also find at this stage that, although the infant cannot effectively visually pursue a stimulus in space, he is beginning to be able to follow his own hand visually. He does this generally by alternating the eyes used as he follows the hand. His visual pursuit of his own hand is his most efficient functional visual act.

The organization at the level of the pons is typified by the first functional movement, the beginning of true reception both auditory and visual, and the generally increased movement.[1]

At about six months of age the infant begins to move into the mid-brain stage of development. The mid-brain consists mainly of the superior and inferior colliculi dorsally and the cerebral peduncles ventrally. Between them is the aqueduct cerebri (Sylvii) which is surrounded ventrally and laterally by the primary nuclei of origin of the occular motor nerves. The fibers of the retina end in the lateral geniculate body (part of the optic thalamus) and the superior colliculus which is part of the mid-brain. These retinal fibers running to the mid-brain are very primitive phylogenetically. In infants they are associated with light and posture. The extraordinary abundance of the sensory nerve supply of the occular muscles and their very intimate connection with the postural centers of the mid-brain are strong indices of the interrelationship of posture, mobility and vision at the mid-brain level. There is, as a result, a very close relationship among eye movements and postural changes, extra occular nerves and labyrinths with concomitant interrelationship of audition and the muscles of the neck and the trunk.[2, 3]

The mid-brain is the area of mediation and integration. By means of the projection fibers of the mid-brain level integration

---

[1]For the purpose of this work the author has not included other sensory and other expressive modalities. For a complete description of those areas and of their related brain level and chronological levels see *Doman-Delacato Developmental Profile,* Copyright the Rehabilitation Center at Philadelphia, 1962.

[2]For an excellent treatment, see Duke Elder, W. S.: *Textbook of Ophthalmology,* St. Louis, Missouri, C. V. Mosby Co., 1946, Vol. I.

[3]Wright, Samson: *Applied Physiology,* 9th Ed., London, Oxford University Press, 1952.

of later functional activity of the cortex can take place. These sub-cortical integrative functions are of far greater importance than are the transcortical associative tracts. For example, if we remove the cortical convolutions which surround the speech areas, we do not produce aphasia because the functional integration of the cortical speech areas take place at a sub-cortical level.[4]

At the mid-brain level we begin to see other relationships to mobility, now for the first time in the third dimension in the form of creeping. This requires audition binaurally, vision binocularly, and the direct relationships of visual fibers, auditory fibers, labyrinth, occulomotor nerves, light and posture reflexes, and the muscles of the neck and trunk, in forming the level of behavior indicated by mylenization and organization at the mid-brain level.

We note at this level a great smoothness and serialization of function. The child creeping at this level does so with great ease and unexcelled efficiency and smoothness. He never again achieves this smoothness of performance on his path toward adulthood. His walking never is as smooth nor as perfectly serialized as he grows toward adulthood.

At the mid-brain level the child becomes a truly land animal. We could wonder if the child is destined to be a quadruped or a biped when observing him at the mid-brain level. This phase of neurological organization is in reality a preparatory phase for making the infant ready for assuming his human upright position when he has achieved all of the functions of the mid-brain level.[5]

The mid-brain child learns to creep. He has achieved the third dimension in movement. He now moves in a cross pattern fashion with the mid-brain as the prime level of neurological organization. He now moves about freely on his hands and knees. His stomach is no longer in contact with the floor. If we observe him closely, we note that his smooth and efficient creeping is

---

[4]For an excellent treatment of these relationships, see Penfield, W., and Roberts, L.: *Speech and Brain Mechanisms*, Princeton Univ. Press, 1959, Chapter 10.
[5]Gesell, Arnold: *The First Five Years of Life*, Harper & Brothers, New York, 1940.

made so because he is now using the *opposite* hand and knee at one time. We note that his right hand and left knee make contact with the floor at the same time and that on the next step the left hand and right knee make contact with the floor. The homolateral pattern of crawling (pons) was typified by using both arm and leg on one side of the body at a time and then alternating the sides. The mid-brain level of mobility (creeping) is in contrast typified by using the arm opposite to the leg used (see Figs. 9 and 10).

The child has now become for the first time able to use functions from both sides of his body in concert.

As the child creeps at the level of mid-brain we note that his environment has expanded significantly and that his whole visual performance has also changed. He now becomes able to use functions from both sides of his body in concert and now

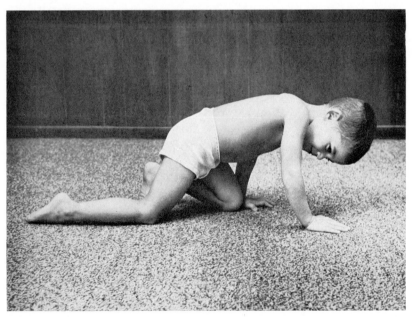

Figure 9. Cross-pattern creeping. This is the first mobility function which requires the use of the opposite arm and leg. Note that as the *right* hand is moved forward the *left* leg moves forward. As this takes place, the head and neck turn slightly toward the *forward* hand.

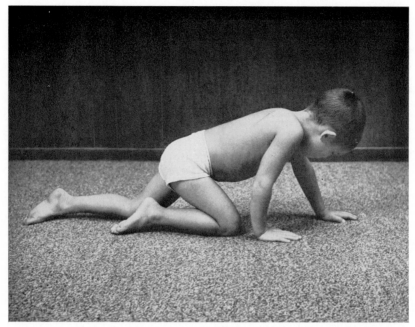

Figure 10. Cross-pattern creeping continues with the opposite phase, as the *left* hand and *right* leg move forward. The head and neck turn toward the *left,* which is the *forward* hand.

becomes able to use both eyes in concert. They become yoked at this stage and begin to look at the same object in space simultaneously. The child has progressed from being *biocular* to being *binocular.*

This is also true of the area of audition. The child at the level of pons does not have the ability to place sounds in space nor does he have a sense of the depth or distance of sound. As he moves into the mid-brain stage he becomes binaural and begins to learn to place sound in space.

The child's hand use comes into greater play at this stage. He develops a prehensile grasp with which he can manipulate objects in space and he learns to follow his hands in space when creeping or when holding an object—using both eyes in concert. Following his own hands in space is the easiest situation for using both eyes at one time. This is the result of the richness of

visual motor nerve supply at this stage and their close relationship with neck and labyrinthian function, which are, in turn,
interrelated to manual function. During this stage a beginning
is made in the ability to follow objects in space binocularly without the added somatic cues of holding the object in the hand.

The most significant changes which take place at this stage
are the increased mobility with the added third dimension and
the added scope of the environment; the change from alternating
one sidedness to crossed two sidedness; the increased efficiency
which is the result of increased smoothness and serialization of
most activity areas; and the new ability to integrate many formerly separated receptive and expressive functions.

We know that diseases affecting the mid-brain affect the ability to be efficiently bilateral. Athetosis and Parkinson's Disease,
both of which have their etiology within the mid-brain, have
symptoms which include inability to creep in a smooth cross-
pattern, inability to be efficiently bilateral, inability to be efficiently binocular, the inability to deal with sound binaurally
and the inability to function in a smooth serialized pattern because of a lack of integration.

At about one year of age the child moves from a mid-brain
type of overall function to early cortical function. Both the
physiology and the topography of the cortex have been so remarkably presented in the literature that the author will deal
only briefly with the physiology of the cortex.[6]

The cortex is responsible for many facets of speech and are
walking. The elementary sensations of touch, pressure, heat and
cold are now mediated by the post central gyrus which receive
the afferent pathways directly. Discrimination between stimuli
and the recognition of objects placed in the hand are probably
associated with the posterior portion of the parietal lobe. These
functions become increasingly functional and stereoagnosis appears.

The visual pathways cross at the optic chasma. This decussation is only partial, both at the cortical level and at the sub-

---

[6]For the most recent and the most authoritative see Penfield, W. and Roberts,
L.: *Speech and Brain Mechanisms*, Princeton, New Jersey, Princeton University
Press, 1959, pp. 1-286.

cortical level, hence, some pathways do not cross over but instead represent the eye on the same side of the brain in which it is located.

The child at this level is becoming increasingly proficient at bilateral activity. He shows much improvement in bilateral control, then begins to experiment with becoming paralateral. He begins to use his hands and arms independently of his feet and legs and masters one of his most human of functions, that of walking.

As he begins to pull himself up on furniture, he begins his first explorations into being a biped. If he has not mastered all of the cross-pattern and bilateral activity of the mid-brain stage, he will not be completely organized neurologically and will not master walking well. The early walking requires that the child move his legs in a cross-pattern. He uses his hands, not in the cross-pattern walking position typical of the well organized older child but instead uses them independently, held above his head or out at his side, serving the purpose of rudders. As the walking becomes more proficient it becomes more bilateral and, by the age of three to four, the child walks in a normal cross-pattern utilizing both his arms and legs for balance and ease of walking. This is refined as he moves toward adulthood (see Fig. 11).

Early cortical hearing begins to be developed when the child begins to use binaural sound stimuli in combination and sounds begin to achieve a stereophonic character. This is the result of the fusion of the two sound receptions received simultaneously by the two ears. It takes place at the level of cortex. It is one of the final acts of readiness for symbolic speech. The child progresses from experimenting with his new world of sound to the speaking of words. He now starts the process of learning both the receptive and expressive components of speech. This process is environmentally completed if the child is neurologically well organized at this point. The child begins to learn the various sound components which are the word names given to things and ideas in his environment. As a result, he learns to speak the language or languages spoken by those around him.

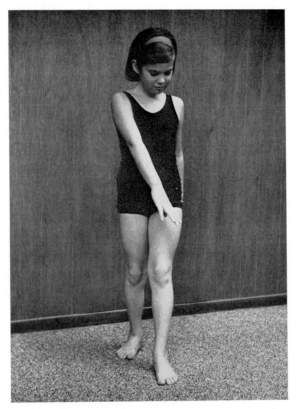

Figure 11. Cross-pattern walking. This is an extension of cross-pattern creeping. Again, the *right* hand and *left* leg move forward with the head and neck turned slightly toward the *forward* hand. Cross-pattern walking is the ideal form of walking, both from a neurological and structural point of view, in that it provides the greatest possible balance for the human when he is upright.

A further sophistication of stereophonic experience is the child's growing fondness for music. This at the outset is bilateral, utilizing both hemispheres of the cortex. Later, as laterality and hemispheric dominance become established, music and tonality in general are relegated to the subdominant hemisphere in well organized individuals, and the skills of sound reception and production which form the skill aspects of human speech become the province of the dominant cortical hemisphere.

At this point we have developed what will become the skilled and the tonal ear. These relate to the dominant and subdominant hemispheres of the cortex. The skilled ear is usually the ear chosen when given a monaural task, such as the watch tick test. The child will usually use the skilled ear for listening to the tick of a clock or to listen to any other one-eared assignment which requires auditory acuity and comprehension. The other ear is usually the ear chosen for turning to a one-eared musical or tonal experience. Both these tests for ascertaining earedness need more investigation relative to reliability, hence are not generally used by the author, excepting in those cases wherein delayed speech or aphasoid characteristics are present. They are used then only as a guide toward the speech performance and not as critical factors in the ascertainment of the dominant-subdominant hemispheric relationship.

The child's visual performance becomes increasingly complex in that he learns to fuse the two separate visual perceptions received by the two eyes into one cortical impression. The end product of this cortical ability to superimpose the two receptions is known as stereopsis. The child can now begin to deal with visual symbols. This is the beginning of the ability to be able to deal with visual abstractions, which is prerequisite to learning how to deal with written letters and words.

One of our great errors in the rearing of children has been the tendency to further accelerate the very rapid development of the first year of life. We find in our culture many parents who push their children toward walking and talking during this already accelerated year of development. As these parents are successful in pushing this development they are no doubt interfering with the ultimate *quality* of neurological organization which the child will achieve. We have seen many children with reading and speech problems who had inadequate neurological organization because they were pushed by parents. For example, we have seen many children who were encouraged to walk long before they were neurologically ready to walk. Since they could not, as a result of the pushing, complete the mid-brain stage of organization they invariably presented some problem of bilaterality, binocularity, general smoothness of coordination, or the inability to integrate receptive or expressive functions well.

In addition, we have caused further qualitative losses in neurological organization culturally by our ignorance of the significance of developmental readiness. We have placed infants in positions and in types of clothing which made it impossible to follow these developmental sequences. We have used play pens to restrict their much needed movement, we have placed them in high chairs and have amused them in lieu of giving them the opportunities needed for proper neurological experiences. We have placed them in clothes and shoes which restrict mobility. Children of creeping age should wear overalls. Their feet should be free so that toes can aid in the creeping function. We have placed them in positions which inhibit bilateral development. These lacks of opportunity for the proper sequential progression through the neurological developmental stages usually result later in some qualitative dysfunction in the development of total neurological organization.

For example, the well-organized 18 month old child is bilateral, binocular and binaural. We have all seen children who did not follow this progression who had some problem in one or more of the areas above. We recently evaluated thirty-two strabismic children whose ages ranged from four to seventeen. We did not record the date of onset of the strabismus. We found that of this group of thirty-two children who were not binocular that twenty-six had chosen to creep very little, or were allowed to creep very little before they walked. It is the opinion of the author that had these children been allowed to creep for an adequate period of time in a proper cross-pattern serialization that many of them would have developed binocularity and would not have become strabismic.[7]

We know that normally children develop binocularity at the mid-brain level. We know further that, if we stimulate the extra occular fibers at the mid-brain level, we can significantly affect eye movements. Such an approach to the treatment of strabismus is not unique. The Optometric Extension Program advocates a

---

[7]See page 150 for results of the treatment of strabismic patients through creeping.

developmental approach to the improvement of binocularity (see page 18).

There are many theories on the development and, therefore the treatment, of strabismus. There is the mechanical theory, the refraction theory, the fusion theory, the positional theory, the innervation theory and the reflex theory, each with its concomitant treatment procedures. The very existence of so many theories with such widely varying biases leads us to believe that we have not found the solution to the treatment of strabismus. The author feels that the most plausible and the most successful concept thus far is that of Keiner, a Dutch ophthalmologist who presents a reflex theory with a developmental bias. It is conceptually in accord with the author's view of the etiology and the treatment of strabismus. The details of treatment are different, however.[8]

Most of the older theories as to the etiology of strabismus are biased toward structure. The author feels strongly that the answer to both diagnosis and treatment lies in a functional approach, as expressed by Keiner and the Optometric Extension Program.

The same is true for the area of audition. We have found that those children, who are not given the opportunity to develop their binaural abilities through adequate experience at the midbrain level, usually find it very difficult to master phonetics in early reading. These are also the children who are seen in many speech clinics as articulation problems. They have not developed adequate receptive binaural skills and, as a result, when called upon to use receptive data in an expressive modality such as in speech or in phonetics, are found to be inadequate.

The milder cases form the great bulk of children in our schools today who do not profit from the teaching of phonetics. Although taught as are the other members of the class, these children are unable to master phonetics. The author feels that this is the result of a lack of complete development of binaural abilities.

---

[8]Keiner, G. B. J.: *New Viewpoints on the Origin of Squint.* A Clinical and Statistical Study on its Nature, Cause and Therapy, The Hague, Martinus Nijhoff Co., 1951, pp. 1-222.

We have also seen the results of the lack of opportunity to develop a proper mobility level. These are the normal children whom we consider incoordinate. We have never established an etiology for their lack of coordination, nor have we resolved the problem. The author feels that these problems also fall within the province of qualitatively poor neurological organization.

From one year of age to 18 months of age the child operates at an early cortical level. The progression of neurological organization now becomes painfully slow, when compared with the explosive growth which took place from birth to one year of age. He needs seven more years to develop from early cortical function to the completion of neurological organization.

The completion of this stage of neurological organization places the child somewhat ahead of the primate. He can now walk bilaterally in a cross-pattern—that is, swinging the opposite arm toward the forward leg and vice versa on the next step. He now has stereopsis, stereophonic hearing and has developed stereoagnosis. He has mastered enough paralateral activity at the cortical level so that he can now oppose his finger and thumb dexterously and, as a result, has fairly sophisticated bilateral manual dexterity and he can supinate and pronate his hand and forearm. These achievements of the young child help him to move about his environment developing greater muscle strength, greater vital capacity and to gain experiences upon which to build later intellectual function.

These are the final vertical achievements possible in neurological organization. Now, after a period of a few years, the child must leave this active bilateral world. He must move on to the next stage of neurological organization—that of laterality—which is unique to man. He has become a truly expressive organism with a spoken language. He must now move on to the stage of a more sophisticated language function, one which includes reading, writing and spelling.

The next step in the progression toward complete human function is the development of cortical hemispheric dominance. Up to this point in cortical function both hemispheres of the cortex operate in concert with a balanced trans-cortical relationship.

Now the two hemispheres begin to develop differentiated functions—one becoming the dominant hemisphere and the other assuming a sub-dominant role. This progression is dictated genetically, hence, right sided parents are apt to have right sided children. Right sided parents who have a genetic bias toward twinning are more apt to have left sided children than if they do not have the twinning bias. *Brain injury or inadequate subcortical organization both result in difficulty in the establishment of hemispheric dominance.* There are many cultural factors which deter the complete establishment of hemispheric dominance. This is especially true for left handed human beings adjusting to our right sided culture.[9]

Sidedness usually begins with hand choice. There is no doubt a genetic bias toward sidedness. We know that there is a high correlation between the inability to establish sidedness and brain injury. As the choice of hand becomes more consistent one notes that the hand becomes more skilled. As a result, its choice is re-enforced. With continued use of a choice hand, either the left or the right, the child begins to develop a choice eye. This is normally the eye on the same side as the choice hand. This is the eye that is closest to the hand and, as a result, is the most convenient eye to use. Continued use further develops the skill of the predominant eye, even though both eyes are being used, one is given preference over the other. With continued use it becomes the stronger eye. The same pattern is true for footedness.

This new trend away from bilaterality and toward consistent single sidedness is unique in man. As it takes place cortical hemispheric function is modified into a dominant-sub-dominant relationship; that is, one hemisphere becomes dominant and controls the skilled side and the other hemisphere is forced to assume a subservient role.

This final lateral development takes place at from five to eight years of age.

---

[9]For greater description see Delacato, C. H.: *The Treatment and Prevention of Reading Problems*, Springfield, Thomas, 1959.

To become totally left sided in a right handed world is difficult. If one evaluates one's surroundings, one finds that most man-made objects are made for the convenience of right sided individuals. Hence, we have left sided individuals constantly battling to maintain the integrity of their left sidedness.

The literature amply corroborates the fact that a significantly large number of stutterers and poor readers are left sided. Mirror writing is fifteen times more common among left handed children than among right handed children.[10]

As sidedness develops, we note a gradual change in tonal and musical activities. The free experimentation with sound changes during the fourth to sixth years to an enjoyment of tonal variations which contain more intrinsic rhythmic patterns and in which rhythm is more obvious. We have all seen children of this age spellbound by a story and then ask to have it re-read and re-read. They enjoy the rhythm of the language. They even enjoy listening to stories which they don't understand at this stage if they are read rhythmically. Children of this age enjoy poetry and choral speaking and anything which has a high rhythmic component. These children cannot help but pay attention to the highly rhythmic television commercials. They are in process of establishing tonal sidedness wherein the dominant cortical hemisphere controls sound skills and the sub-dominant hemisphere controls the tonal activity. Stutterers never make this tonal adjustment, hence they stutter. They are caught at mid-point of organization with both cortical hemispheres in balance and, therefore, in conflict. If we artificially resolve the balance by having one hemisphere become dominant the stutter disappears. This is why stutterers cannot stutter when singing and why they rarely stutter when reading rhythmic poetry or performing in choral speech.

This final lateral progression of neurological organization results in a totally-human human being who is right handed, right eyed and right footed with the left hemisphere of the brain controlling the skills, and the right hemisphere of the brain assum-

---

[10]Gates, R. R.: *Human Genetics*, New York, MacMillan Co., 1946. Vol. II, p. 1161.

ing a sub-dominant role and being the seat of tonality; or a left handed, left eyed and left footed human being whose right cortical hemisphere controls the skills and whose left cortical hemisphere becomes sub-dominant and becomes the seat of tonality.

This final lateral progression begins at about the age of three and is almost complete by the age of seven. It normally is totally complete by the age of eight.

We can corroborate the progress of neurological organization clinically. The mobility functions of growing and maturing children indicate the level of neurological organization they have reached. There are many other indices. They become less hyperactive as they grow older, they learn with greater facility, indeed they generally follow the patterns outlined by Gesell in all of his studies. These changes in behavior, which Gesell put into the literature and to which many others have added, now make up the body of knowledge known as child development. There is complete agreement that these changes are the result of changes which take place within the child.

A more mechanical measurement of the process of neurological organization can be made by the electro-encephalogram.

The electro-encephalogram changes in children from birth on. It begins as a disorganized morass and ends as fairly organized in normal children at about age eight, when laterality has been completely established. The electro-encephalogram of the new born is a jumbled mass. It has no rhythm. At one month rhythm appears if one places the electrodes over the primary visual areas. The rhythm fits into a frequency of three per second with a somewhat larger amplitude between the crest and the trough of the waves.

From this point there is a gradual increase in the rhythmicity of the electro-encephalogram. The frequency of the waves increases gradually to four to seven waves per second. There is also a gradual decrease in the amplitude of the waves.

At about the eighth birthday (when cortical hemispheric dominance is completely established) the rhythm becomes quite stable. There are about ten waves per second (alpha waves) from this time through adulthood. The pattern is organized and the

amplitude of the waves is predictable enough to be used diagnostically.

As we view this ontogenetic progression chronologically, we
find that the first year of life takes us rapidly up to the level of
cortex and that the progression of neurological organization then
decelerates dramatically. We have erroneously tried to further
accelerate the development of the first year of life by encouraging the activities which we feel are human, such as walking and
talking. In addition, we have neglected to give to some of our
children the opportunities to take full advantage of each hour
of this highly accelerated developmental year by restricting
their ability to crawl and to creep for a long enough period of
time prior to moving on to the next stage.

We are compounding these errors by not helping children during the very slow moving progression of ages one to eight. We
should help them toward complete bilaterality during the early
part of this stage. We should then help them toward complete
humanity by watching to see what they begin to develop as a
choice side. We should then help them to develop that sidedness exclusively. Here is the area in which children can be accelerated toward more complete neurological organization.[11]

If we juxtapose the phylogenetic development of the nervous
system and its significant functions with the ontogenetic development of a single human being, on its course toward neurological
organization resulting in speech and reading, we find some interesting relationships.

As we study these relationships it becomes apparent immediately that the organizational factor exclusive to man is the establishment of cortical hemispheric dominance and, also, that man
is the only creature who can speak, read and write.

	Highest Neurological Level	Mobility	Vision	Audition
Newborn Infant	Medulla	Trunkal Mvmt	Reflex	Reflex
Fish	Medulla	Trunkal Mvmt	Reflex	Reflex
Four month old Infant	Pons	Homolateral Crawling	Bi-ocular	Bi-aural

[11]For greater detail see Delacato, C.: *The Treatment and Prevention of Reading
Problems,* Springfield, Thomas, 1959.

	Highest Neurological Level	Mobility	Vision	Audition
Amphibian	Pons	Homolateral Crawling	Bi-ocular	Bi-aural
Ten month old Infant	Mid-brain	Cross-pattern Creeping	Binocular Yoking	Binaural
Reptile	Mid-brain	Cross-pattern Creeping	Binocular Yoking	Binaural
One year old Infant	Early Cortex	Crude Walking	Early Fusion	Early Stereophonic
Primate	Early Cortex	Crude Walking	Early Fusion	Early Stereophonic
Eight year old (who speaks, reads and writes)	Cortical Hemispheric Dominance	Cross-pattern Walking	Stereopsis with predominant eye	Stereophonic hearing with predominant ear

Chapter 6

NEUROLOGICAL ORGANIZATION AND
BRAIN INJURY

Since it has been impossible in the past to see these developmental phases in a mass situation because of the great speed
with which they are achieved during the first year of life and
the very slow pace in which they are achieved during the subsequent seven years of life, we have had difficulty in ascertaining the *significance* of normal developmental progressions. In
addition, we have never been able to relate these developmental
processes to neurology and neurological development because
we have never had neurological data on the normal children we
have observed. Gesell, through his monumental work, has given
us many insights into normal development but he too was handi-
capped by the vagaries of chronology and by the total lack of
adequate neurological data. As a result, there does not exist in
the literature a study of child development wherein the developmental data was correlated with actual neurological physiology.

The author, with his co-workers at the Rehabilitation Center
at Philadelphia, conducted a study aimed at overcoming these
two historical weaknesses.

We studied seventy-six severely brain injured children. Because they were severely brain injured, the vagaries of chronology were not present since all of the children were significantly
retarded developmentally. As a result, their natural progression
toward complete neurological organization was extremely slow
and in most cases it was highly questionable whether complete
neurological organization could ever be achieved. By using such
a group we had overcome chronological variations and had sub-

stituted extremely slow or non-existent developmental progression.

In addition, our subjects, since they were all severely brain injured, had all been throughly evaluated neurologically, hence, we were dealing in each case with known pathology. This group presented to us, therefore, both a predictable developmental chronology moving in painfully slow motion, and also known pathology. In the past, neither of these had been achieved *together* in dealing with a universal rationale for human development as related to known neurophysiology.

As we arrived at a developmental lag in the area of mobility, we passively imposed that movement pattern upon the body of each child to see whether working from function to structure would give us developmental-neurological co-relations, and whether working from function to structure would result in a significant change in the chronological-developmental mobility retardation which each child exhibited.

Children With Severe Brain Injuries (Neurological Organization in Terms of Mobility)[1]

The large number of conferences, seminars, and publications regarding the brain-injured child indicates not so much the volume of new information available but rather the intensity of the search for new information.

We had long been dissatisfied with the results of our own methods of treatment and believed that the time requirements in treating children with severe brain injuries could scarcely be justified in light of the low percentage of marked successes as compared with children who were essentially without treatment.

During 1956 and 1957 we developed a new approach to such cases, the goal of which was to establish in brain-injured children the developmental stages observed in normal children. The program which aimed at both normal and damaged brain levels consisted of (*a*) permitting the child normal develop-

[1]Doman, R., Spitz, E., Zucman, E., Delacato, C., and Doman, G.: *J. A. M. A.*, *174*:257-262, Sept., 1960. Initial Summary, Tables, Charts, Photographs, and Bibliography of the original article are not included. This article is reprinted through the permission of the American Medical Association.

mental opportunities in areas in which the responsible brain level was undamaged; (*b*) externally imposing the bodily patterns of activity which were the responsibility of damaged brain levels; and (*c*) utilizing additional factors to enhance neurological organization.

The team used consisted of a physiatrist, a neurosurgeon, an orthopedic surgeon, a nurse, a physical therapist, and a psychologist. In 1958, a two-year outpatient study was begun which used these developmental stages in the treatment of seventy-six brain-injured children. Each patient was seen bimonthly.

MATERIAL

Subjects.—This study of seventy-six children includes every child seen in the Children's Clinic during the study period who met the following criteria: 1. The existence of brain injury. (For the purpose of this study, brain-injured children are defined as those children whose lesion lies in the brain. The definition includes both traumatic and nontraumatic lesions but excludes children who are genetically defective.) 2. A minimum of six months' treatment. 3. No child was eliminated because of the severity of his involvement.

Diagnosis of Brain Pathology.—The diagnosis was made after neurological examination and, in most patients, after an EEG, air study, and subdural tap had been done. The group of seventy-six was composed of children who had spasms, athetosis, ataxia, rigidities, tremors, and mixed symptoms; twenty-four of these children had clinical seizures.

Classification of Brain Pathology.—The brain pathology was classified as to type, location, and degree in the following manner.

1. Type: (*a*) unilateral brain damage: This group contained fifteen children with either subdural hematoma (all operated on), vascular malformation, or hemiatrophy of nonspecific causation. Of these fifteen children, four had hemispherectomies performed by us. (*b*) bilateral brain damage: This group contained sixty-one children with conditions such as hydrocephalus, subdural hematoma (all operated on), kernicterus, postencephalitic damage, dysgenesis of corpus callosum, dysgenesis of cerebellum, dysgenesis of cortex, porencephaly, or diffuse cortical atrophy of nonspecific causation. We per-

formed fourteen ventriculojugular and two ventriculoperitoneal shunts on the sixteen hydrocephalic patients. The therapeutic program was instituted no sooner than ten months after surgery.

2. Location: Upon air study, thirty children demonstrated dilatation of the lateral ventricles, and twelve demonstrated dilatation of the entire ventricular system, thus indicating the presence of subcortical as well as cortical damage. Locating these lesions in terms of the Phelps-Fay classification, there were sixty-one cerebral lesions (spastic patients), twelve midbrain lesions (athetoid patients), three basal ganglion lesions (two patients with tremor, one with rigidity), and ten cerebellar lesions (ataxic patients).

3. Degree: Both clinical examination and neurosurgical diagnostic procedures indicated that the degree of brain damage ranged from mild to severe. No child was eliminated from this study due to severity of either clinical symptoms or degree of brain pathology.

Age at Beginning of Study.—The ages ranged from twelve months to nine years, with a median age of twenty-six months and a mean age of thirty months. The children were separated into three age groups of developmental significance: 0-18 months, sixteen children; eighteen to thirty-six months, forty-one children; and over thirty-six months, nineteen children.

Level and Stages of Movement at Beginning of Therapy.— The level of movement was defined according to a modification of the developmental patterns of Gesell and co-workers and Fay, and these were numerically designated for reference purposes. The stages described are (*a*) moving arms and legs without forward movements, (*b*) crawling, (*c*) creeping, and (*d*) walking. In our experience, each stage described was dependent on the successful completion of the previous stage.

IQ, Affect, and Speech.—No child was eliminated because of severity of deficiency in these areas.

Duration of Treatment.—The duration of treatment ranged from six to twenty months, with a mean of eleven months.

METHOD

After thorough neurological studies, the children were evaluated to determine their disabilities in functional terms. An outpatient program of neurological organization was then pre-

scribed and taught to the parents. The parents were required
to carry out the program exactly as prescribed. The children's
course was reviewed by the team on an average of every two
months, and treatment changes were made to correspond to
new developmental levels of accomplishment. The treatment
consisted of two types.

Treatment Type I.—All nonwalking children (56) were required to spend all day on the floor in the prone position and
were encouraged to crawl (prone method) or creep (hand-
knee method) when that level of accomplishment was possible.
The only permissible exceptions were to feed, love, and treat
the child. This increased the opportunity for the reproduction
of the normal functional-positional situation of a healthy child
during the first thirteen months of life.

Treatment Type II.—In each case, at that level of accomplishment at which pathology precluded the child's advancement to the next developmental stage, a specific pattern of
activity was prescribed which passively imposed on the central
nervous system the functional activity which was normally the
responsibility of that damaged brain level. Initially these patterns were in some cases partially, and in other cases completely, those which had been described by Fay. As time
passed, our team discontinued some of these, modified others,
and added those which it believed to be useful. Each of these
patterns had its counterpart in the normal developmental
growth of a healthy child so well described by Gesell and
Amatruda. The children were patterned for five minutes, four
times daily, seven days a week without exception. The patterns were administered by three adults. One adult turned
the head, another moved the right arm and leg, and the third
moved the left arm and leg. The patterns were to be performed smoothly and rhythmically at all levels.

Activity Pattern I (Homolateral): Children who could not
crawl and those who crawled below cross-pattern level were
patterned in the homolateral pattern, which was accomplished
by one adult turning the head while the adult on the side to
which the head was turned flexed the arm and leg. The adult
on the opposite side extended both limbs. As the head was
turned, the flexed limbs extended while the extended limbs
flexed.

Activity Pattern II (Cross-Pattern): Children who could crawl in cross-pattern or who could creep were patterned in cross-pattern, which was accomplished by one adult turning the head, while the adult on the side toward which the head was turned flexed the arm and extended the leg, the adult on the opposite side extended the arm and flexed the leg. When the head was turned, the position of the limbs was reversed.

Activity Pattern III (Cross-Pattern): Children who walked but poorly were also patterned at the cross-pattern level.

Treatment for Neurological Organization.—To enhance neurological organization, the children were evaluated in the light of the functions described below, and a treatment program was devised. The program included the following stages: 1. When tests showed sensory losses or when results of tests were indefinite due to communication problems, the children were placed on a program of sensory stimulation which included application of heat and cold, brushing, pinching, and establishment of body image appreciation by letting the child experience the relationship between his hand and his face, his hand and his mother's face, and similar relationships. 2. As each child reached the point where laterality influenced neurological organization, a program to establish dominance was instituted. 3. A breathing program to improve vital capacity was prescribed. All other therapy and use of mechanical aids were discontinued, except for anticonvulsant medication when indicated.

RESULTS

The results were evaluated according to the following categories: (1) global results; (2) results in the light of chronological age; (3) results in the light of the individual disposition of each patient; and (4) results in the light of the functional level at the onset of the program.

Global Results.—The mean improvement of mobility was 4.2 levels. The mean level of mobility was 4.4 at the beginning of the program and 8.6 at the end of the program. The range of improvement was 0 to 12 levels. If we consider perfect walking the potential for every child, the group achieved 51 per cent of this goal.

The following findings are of interest: Of the twenty children unable to move and the seventeen unable to walk, none remained at these stages. Twelve children were ready to walk at the end of the study. Eight were creeping cross-pattern (level 10), and four were holding onto objects (level 11).

Eight of the group who could walk initially improved significantly in their walking but did not become perfect and, therefore, could not be considered as having increased their functional competence by one level. All but two of the other children improved by one or more levels.

Eleven children learned to walk completely independently. All but two of these had begun treatment at, or before, two years of age, and all achieved completely independent walking in less than twelve months of treatment. The functional level of this group at the beginning of the study was virtually the same as the level of the other sixty-five children. The entire group mean level at the outset was 4.4, compared with a mean of 4.1 for this group of eleven who learned to walk independently.

Only six children were discharged, all of whom had learned to walk perfectly; three of these had been walking poorly and three had been unable to walk at the beginning of the program. The other eight who had learned to walk and the other seventeen who had improved in walking were not discharged because of residual problems in speech or behavior.

Results in Light of Chronological Age.—The children were separated into three age groups of developmental significance for purposes of evaluation. There was no significant difference of mean improvement among the three different age groups.

Individual Results in Light of Functional Level at Beginning of Study.—An analysis of the original level—ultimate level disposition of each case indicates an over-all improvement of 4.1 levels within the study.

Rate of Improvement in Light of Functional Level at Beginning of Study.— The levels of improvement were evaluated by analysis of thirteen levels in terms of functional components.

COMMENT

We found significant improvement when we compared the results of the classic procedures we had previously followed with the results of the procedures described above. It is our opinion that the significance of the difference tends to corroborate the validity of the hypothesis set up as the theoretical basis of the program.

These procedures are based on the premise that certain brain levels, i.e., pons, midbrain, and cortex, have separate, consecutive responsibilities in terms of mobility. The goal of these procedures (neurological organization) is to create a climate in which a brain-injured child may develop and utilize those brain levels which are uninjured as they are developed in the normal child concurrent with myelinization during the first eighteen months of life.

We have observed that the opportunities to crawl and creep are rarely accorded to the brain-injured child. Great emphasis should be placed on permitting the brain-injured child to remain on the floor, which Gesell and co-workers have described as the normal child's "athletic field," thus giving the child an opportunity to utilize and exploit uninjured brain levels and achieve the functions for which such brain levels are responsible.

After neurological examination and testing had established the level of brain injury, we imposed on the child's central nervous system patterns of activity which have as their goal the reproduction of normal activities which would have been the product of the injured brain level had it not been injured. The pattern aspect of the procedure was achieved after a study and modification of Fay's work with the brain-injured child and Gesell's work with the normal child and was then integrated into the procedure developed by us.

It is our opinion that, to be successful in such a program, the procedure must be carried out "wholistically." While we placed varying emphasis upon the importance of different areas within the program, it was our experience that success could not be achieved by using the components of the program in isolation.

We believe that the program must include (*a*) the opportunity for the brain-injured child to spend prolonged periods on the floor in the prone or quadruped position, so that he may crawl or creep in order to utilize uninjured brain areas in physiological development. Given this opportunity, the brain-injured child may advance several developmental levels unaided; (*b*) the utilization of patterns of activity administered passively to a child which reproduce the mobility functions for which injured brain levels are responsible; (c) a program of sensory stimulation to make the child body-conscious in terms of position sense and proprioception. We believe that sensory reception is a prerequisite to motor expression; (d) a program of establishing cortical hemispheric dominance through the development of unilateral handedness, footedness, and "eyedness." This was instituted when a lack of neurological organization at this level so indicated; and (e) the institution of a breathing program to achieve the maximal vital capacity, since, in our experience, we had observed the restricted vital capacity and the recurrence of respiratory difficulties in many brain-injured children.

While we think that this program resulted in benefits to the children studied in the areas of language and affect, we confined this report to results achieved in terms of mobility. A later report will deal with the results achieved in other areas by this program of neurological organization.

We wish to stress the fact that no child was eliminated from the study due to initial lack of affect or mobility. It can be observed from the facts presented that many of the children, when initially evaluated, showed little affect and no mobility, and that a large number of them made significant progress. It should also be stressed that during the study all other programs of therapy or habilitation were discontinued and that no mechanical aids, such as braces or crutches, were used.

We place emphasis upon the fact that the children studied were evaluated and treated with reference to the central neurological lesion rather than upon the symptomatic results of the central lesion.

It is our opinion that the results of this study, when compared with the results of our previous work, are sufficiently encouraging to warrant an expanded and continued study of these procedures.

We do not believe that all the techniques which would be useful in achieving neurological organization have been developed by this study. We think that many additional techniques may be developed which would speed the process of habilitation of children with severe brain injuries and perhaps increase the number of types of brain injuries which can be treated. Later reports will deal with the results of studies being conducted at the time of writing.

SUMMARY

A two year study was conducted on seventy-six brain-injured children. Its goal was to determine whether a program aimed at neurological organization would be productive of greater results in terms of mobility than we had previously achieved by more classic therapy.

The children studied were both evaluated and treated in light of their central neurological lesions in a program which we had devised to utilize undamaged brain levels to achieve the physiological functions for which such levels are responsible and to assist children at damaged brain levels in achieving function, as far as possible, by means of a program designed to reproduce normal activity. The preliminary results of this study are encouraging. Further studies of these procedures will be undertaken.

The speech results of the above study were not included in the article because the article dealt primarily with mobility results rather than language growth. Each child was evaluated in speech prior to the program. *No speech therapy was given to any child during the program.*

The children who could not speak at the beginning of the program and who were old enough chronologically and, therefore, should have been speaking at that time, were designated as retarded in speech. Of these retarded children who did not speak, 59 per cent began to speak words at some time during the program even though there was no speech therapy nor any effort made to encourage them to speak during the program. We feel that the onset of speech was the direct result of enhanced neurological organization.

To Recapitulate

Man has evolved phylogenetically in a known pattern. The ontogenetic development of normal humans in general recapitulates that phylogenetic process. We have been able to take children who deviated from normal development (severely brain injured) and through the extrinsic imposition of normal patterns

of movement and behavior have been able to neurologically organize them sufficiently so that they could be placed within the
human developmental pattern of crawling, creeping and walking.
Finally, with man's unique lateral neurological function added to
this structure, talking, reading and writing developed.

If we can accomplish this with the severely brain injured, we
should be able to organize those children who are not brain injured, but are only neurologically disorganized, with much
greater results and with much less effort.

Chapter 7

DIAGNOSTIC PROCEDURE

THE DIAGNOSTIC procedure should proceed from sub-cortical levels to cortical levels, and then to laterality. This is the most logical procedure since it sequentially retraces the course of neurological organization and also represents the sequence of treatment.

It is very important to have the communication problem discussed and understood fully. The author has found that there are varied definitions in the minds of parents of emotionally toned descriptive words such as, stammering, stuttering, nonreader, poor reader, retarded reader, or word blind. These distorted definitions result in faulty understanding and, in some instances, in faulty acceptance of the symptoms by parents. It is also rare, indeed, to have the referring agency, clinic or school make a complete enough evaluation so that the symptoms are fully stated or understood. An understanding of the symptoms is extremely important, for example: We see brain injured children who are completely word blind in reading but who have normal speech. We must conclude that this is the result of sub-cortical lesion, for injuries to the cortex affect language and speech as a whole (posterior lesions affecting reception, anterior lesions affecting expression).[1]

A further clarification of symptoms is the use of standardized tests for reading and spelling. There are a number of such tests which are both diagnostic and analytic in nature. Such test scores should always be compared with results in arithmetic to

---

[1]Wright, S: *Applied Physiology*, Ninth Ed., London, Oxford Univ. Press, 1952, p. 655.

ascertain if there is a difference in performance between the language and mathematical areas. If there is not such a difference, one must suspect an intellectual limitation as the possible etiological factor.

The use of Intelligence Test results is helpful at this stage. The author favors the Wechsler Intelligence Scale for Children, in that it not only gives a verbal I. Q. (which is invalidated in great part by the existence of a language problem) but it also gives a performance I. Q. with which the verbal performance can be compared.

From the above we can assess the problem, assess present performance and can, in light of intelligence, ascertain the potential for performance.

We now proceed with the history questionnaire in search of possible etiological factors which might, in turn, lead us to greater clarification of the problem and toward greater diagnostic validity. These questions should be asked of the parents with the child not present.

CONDITIONS DURING PREGNANCY

The questioning should be aimed at eliciting any factors which might be related to etiology. The presence of spotting, measles, illness on the part of the mother, great weight gain, severe infections or high temperatures, traumatic incidents, R.H. factors and gross discomfort throughout pregnancy might be significant.

CONDITIONS AT BIRTH

The questioning should be aimed at eliciting possible traumatic factors. Severity of labor, length of labor, whether it was the mother's first labor, type and amount of anaesthesia used, type of presentation, and instruments used are all important to the ascertainment of a possible hypoxia or a possible frank birth trauma. The mother should be questioned about the condition of the baby immediately at birth. If she was not conscious, the birth notes are many times helpful. The immediacy of the birth cry is of prime consideration.

EARLY DEVELOPMENT AND CHILDHOOD DISEASES

The questioning should be aimed at eliciting responses relative to the early vitality of the newborn. Early strength of sucking and early activity levels are important indices of possible trauma. Question carefully the feeding, sleep and elimination during the first six months of life. The number of childhood diseases is sometimes a further indication of vitality. The most important aspect of early childhood diseases is temperature. Prolonged high temperatures and unexpected and unexplainable spiking of temperatures are sometimes indices of trauma.

MOBILITY AND ACTIVITY LEVELS DURING FIRST SIX MONTHS

The questioning should be aimed at determining the opportunity for mobility which was given the infant and the amount of mobility actually demonstrated by the infant. If necessary, have the parent describe in chronological detail a typical day for the child. This will help in the evaluation of the opportunity afforded the child to move. Great lethargy or constant motion are possible indices of trauma or faulty organization.

ONSET AND DEGREE OF CRAWLING

The questioning should be aimed at ascertaining the age of onset of crawling and the quality of the crawling, if possible. The time for the onset of crawling is apt to be unreliable unless the parent refers to a pediatric record or a baby book. Since parents are not generally cognizant of a qualitative factor in crawling, the most qualitative evaluation which can usually be secured is whether the child moved in any fashion which seemed strange to the mother.

ONSET AND QUALITY OF CREEPING

Ascertaining the onset of creeping is difficult without referring to records. The questioning should be aimed at ascertaining the number of weeks which the child spent creeping. Although the parent will not usually be familiar with the qualitative aspects of creeping, she will usually remember if there was anything unusual about the mobility function, such as rolling over to achieve mobility, sliding on the buttocks to achieve mobility, using the arms but dragging the feet while moving or creeping on hands and feet instead of on hands and knees.

It is very helpful at this point to ask for a typical daily schedule so that the overall activity level can be assessed. Look for the tendency to be too restrictive in clothing, sleep schedule and in area allowed for movement, such as over-confinement to a playpen. Ask about climbing. The tendency to early climbing and to a great deal of climbing leads us to question the amount of creeping in which the child engaged.

AGE OF WALKING

Ascertain this from written records if possible. Question to find out whether the infant was encouraged to walk, given a walker, or whether he spent much time holding on to the edge of the playpen and walking. Ascertain whether the early walking was fraught with unnecessary falls and whether it was unusual in any way, such as walking on the toes, very fast walking, very slow walking, constantly tilted to one side or very belabored.

AGE OF TALKING

The questions should be aimed at uncovering the child's history of dealing with sounds. Through records, if possible, find the age of the child when he began to speak words and sentences. Check for a history of articulation difficulties and ascertain whether the child has gone through developmental stammering or stuttering.

Ask about the quality of communication and the speed with which words flow. Ascertain whether there is normal voice inflection and whether there is facial distortion during speech.

TRAUMATIC INJURIES

List all of the childhood diseases with special emphasis on the degree and length of temperature. List all accidents and use of anaesthesia, with special emphasis on head injuries, unconsciousness, seizure type episodes and any possible anoxic or hypoxic situations.

List all injuries to eyes, hands, arms and legs. Find the exact ages at which they took place and the degree of trauma. It is important to ascertain how long the trauma persisted, such as eye patching, splinting and casting. A broken arm at the age of creeping or at the age of beginning writing many times interferes significantly with subsequent neurological organization.

SLEEP PATTERN

Ask the parent to observe the child while he is sleeping. If the child sleeps in either one of the positions below we can assume that he is well organized at the level of pons (see Figs. 7 and 8).[2]

If the child does not sleep in one of these positions, have the parent turn the child's head to the opposite direction from which it is facing while the child is asleep. *One of the following should take place if the child is well organized at the level of Pons.*

     1. As the head is turned the body configuration should reverse itself and the child should remain asleep.

     2. As the head is turned the child should resist its turning and should return it to its original position and the child should remain asleep.

     3. The child should awaken.

If the child allows his head to be turned and if his body configuration does not change and, if he does not awaken, we can assume that he is not well organized at the level of pons. We ascertain this level of organization during sleep while the higher neural centers are not functioning suppressively on this vestigial reflex synergy.

TONALITY

We can ascertain the tonal abilities of the child roughly by questioning general practices with music, such as listening to radio, records, and school music and instrumental participation. We can also ask the child whether he enjoys music and we can

---

[2]For other pictures and greater detail see Delacato, C. H.: *The Treatment and Prevention of Reading Problems*, Springfield, Thomas, 1959.

ask both the parents and his school how well he performs in music. For a further test, in a school situation, we can administer one of the musical aptitude tests given in schools today.

We find that upwards of 90 per cent of our cases who cannot establish cortical hemispheric dominance perform above the mean in music. This is probably the result of their inability to lateralize. As a result, they try hard to establish dominance and, since tonality is with them earlier, and since it requires less skill, they attempt to make both hemispheres tonal or subdominant in nature. The remaining small percentage of our cases are usually extremely poor on tonal performance, most of them verge on being monotones and dislike any form of music. These children have made the opposite adjustment. In striving to establish laterality they strive to make both hemispheres skilled and attempt to negate the tonal aspects of language. This small group is generally highly motivated.

As a result of the original parent interview we can clearly, but tentatively, define the problem and we can garner some possible etiological avenues for further investigation. Those areas in which there is a strong possibility of etiology should be referred for consultation and further study.

We now move on to the clinical evaluation of the child. The purposes of the clinical evaluation are:

1. To ascertain whether there is a lack of neurological organization present.
2. To ascertain the specific levels at which neurological organization is lacking.
3. To establish a basal level of organization, that is, the highest level of neurological organization which has been achieved. The basal level of neurological organization is the level at which treatment must begin.

The child's overall coordination should be observed. Watch him move about to see whether he moves smoothly and efficiently. Does he resemble other children of his own age in his movement patterns? Does he make excessive noise as he moves about? Does he move constantly? Is he hyperactive? Is he placid? Observe his general reactions to his environment.

Look for indices of perceptual confusions. Does he bump into things? Does he appear careless or clumsy? Does he handle things with his hands well or does he overshoot his targets? Does he expend the normal amount of effort in his interactions?

Observe his head and body positions. If he pulls his chin in too far, or if he thrusts it out too far, or if he holds his head to one side or another, all may be indications of faulty visual or perceptual relationships.

Most children, seen by clinics or schools for speech or reading problems, vary from having some mobility to having good mobility, hence the use of the clinical evaluations for mobility at the spinal cord and medulla areas is rare. With most children we see we can assume that they have the simple trunkal movements which are the province of the spinal cord and the medulla. In those cases of very severe brain injury, where the child is so severely disabled that he tends to be immobile, we evaluate very basic spinal cord and medulla mobility functions.

The procedure is to have the child attempt to move its body while in the prone and supine positions while the head is stabilized (held by the examiner) at mid-point. The child should be able to move his body in an undulating fish-like manner. Additionally, all of the typical procedures for the ascertainment of possible spinal cord lesions are used, such as testing sensation of lower limbs for heat, cold, touch, deep touch, pain, pressure and kinaesthesia. The typical application of the Babinski and Marie-Foix reflexes are also helpful diagnostically at this level. It is impossible to have children with such a low level of function in a normal school situation. Such children are seen, however, in neurosurgical clinics, hospitals and rehabilitation centers.

The next higher level is that of the pons. In children who have considerable mobility it is difficult to evaluate the existence of the tonic neck reflex, which is a function of the pons because higher levels of neurological organization supercede the function of the pons. The tonic neck reflex remains only as a vestigial reflex. One procedure is to ask the child to crawl on the floor with his stomach in constant contact with the floor. It is difficult to elicit a pure response because higher levels of function tend to interfere and the crawling becomes an unreliable indication of organization at this level.

The author has found that the ascertainment of the presence of neurological organization at the level of pons is most reliably and most validly accomplished while the child is asleep. Evaluating the child while he is asleep precludes interference of higher levels. For procedure see page 83.

At this level we also observe the child visually. A child who has not moved past this level of organization visually will exhibit an alternating strabismus. He will look at a visual stimulus first with one eye while suppressing the other and then will reverse the procedure. This can be observed by asking the child to visually pursue an object. While the child is doing so, the examiner should look at the eyes. The alternating strabismus is readily observed.

Children at this level are able to respond to the sound of the human voice. They should be able to turn accurately toward an oral stimulus and they should do so efficiently and without hesitation.

The author wishes to state as this time that a lack of organization at the level of spinal cord, medulla, and pons are relatively rarely found in children who can walk without aid and who are not frankly brain injured. *Children who are not organized at these low levels are usually severely disabled.*

The next level of evaluation is the mid-brain level. At this level we see many children who are "normal" but who are very poorly organized. The great majority of the children seen by the author for problems of speech or reading present some inadequacy of neurological organization at the level of mid-brain.

We proceed by asking the child to creep on the floor on his hands and knees. He should do so in the fashion which is typical for the normal nine month old infant—in cross-pattern. His opposite hand and foot should strike the floor simultaneously and his head should turn slightly toward his forward hand. This process should be reversed for the next step. The hands should be palm down and flat and the fingers should be pointing straight ahead. The whole process should be smooth and synergistic (see Figs. 9 and 10).

Any deviation from this pattern is an indication of a lack of organization at this level. For a further clarification of cross pattern creeping the author suggests that the reader spend some time observing a typical nine month old infant creep about. The reader will be struck with the obvious universality of the factors making up cross pattern creeping and will also be struck with the great efficiency and striking spontaneity of a perfect cross-pattern in creeping.

A child who is well organized at the level of mid-brain has a yoking of the two eyes. By observing the eyes one can readily observe if they are functioning in concert. This can be ascertained by having the subject fixate on a target and by projecting a beam of light from the side toward the eyes. In eyes which are yoked and which are functioning in concert the beam of light will be reflected in the eyes at the same distance from each of the pupils. If there is further question relative to the eyes functioning in concert, the cover test can be used. Have the child fixate the bridge of the examiner's nose. Cover one of the child's eyes with your hand. After ten seconds uncover the eye. As you uncover the eye observe it to see how much lateral or vertical adjustment it makes when uncovered. Repeat the process for the other eye. Repeat the process for both eyes while having the child fixate on an object at far point. If the adjustment of the covered eye is obvious as it is uncovered, the child is probably not using his eyes in concert and there is raised a question relative to the quality and strength of his ability to fuse.

Children at this level should be able to react to gestural and tonal directions. They should be able to produce all of the sound components which make up their native language and should do so spontaneously.

The next level of evaluation is the level of early cortex. We first evaluate the mobility which is at this level cross pattern walking. Ask the child to walk, preferably in a goal-directed situation, to reduce consciousness of the walking. The walking should be executed in a smooth cross-pattern. As the child's right foot moves forward his left arm should move forward. They should both move forward in a smooth pattern and the left hand should point slightly toward the right foot. The process should be reversed on the next step. The left foot and right arm move forward and the right hand points slightly at the left foot (see Fig. 12).

The opposite arm and leg should function in a smooth, constant reciprocal pattern.

Children with language problems have historically been categorized as poorly coordinated. If one observes such children closely, one sees a lack of patterning in their walking. They tend to use the arm and leg on the same side of the body at one time for moving forward. They tend to walk in a one-sided pattern

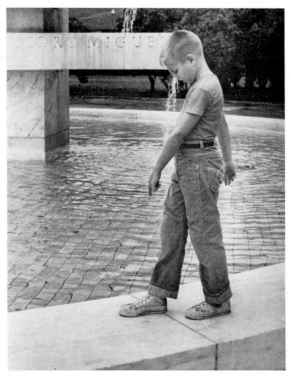

Figure 12. Note the increased balance which results and the turning of the head and neck. (Courtesy James Wolf, Coordinator, Special Education, Panama, Canal Zone.)

typical of the primate. One can readily see that a one-sided walking pattern is most inefficient and that, if one were to run in such a pattern he would be in constant danger of falling, for he has no reciprocal motion to keep him in balance.

We next evaluate the child's ability to supinate and to pronate. We ask him to hold out his hands while the elbows are bent and ask him to turn his palms up and down repeatedly. A slow performance of this task is an indication of poor organization at this level.

We also evaluate his ability to oppose his thumb and his forefinger. He should be able to do this smoothly and without great effort at this level. There should be no significant difference between the two hands in the performance of these two tasks, if the child is well organized at this level.

We next evaluate the child's overall general affective performance. The well organized child at this level should be able to play with all of the toys and playground equipment found in the typical nursery school. He should be proficient in and should enjoy much physical activity and should be gaining the proper caution of dangers in his physical environment.

At this juncture of development the child should be able to pass a functional visual evaluation. We have been naive in the past in evaluating visual functions. We have been structurally oriented, hence, we have looked for structural deviations of the eye. We have also been erroneous in considering acuity as the most significant visual factor. The old days of evaluating the eyes for acuity, one at a time, are gone. The author has seen many children who pass such a monocular acuity test for each eye and have total suppression when the two eyes are used simultaneously. Testing the eyes one at a time is a structural approach which cannot be valid because the use of the two eyes is a learned process, hence, it is functional and is dependent on developmental variants. The child at this level should be able to pass a valid binocular evaluation of visual functions given by a visual specialist who is cognizant of the developmental aspects of vision. *He should not test the eyes, he should test the vision.* His visual evaluation should include visual fields, imbalance tests, both lateral and vertical at far and near points; fusion, fusion ranges, stereopsis, accommodation, convergence, the balance between accommodation and convergence, simultaneousness of vision, and acuity for each eye while the tested eye is perceiving the target and the non-tested eye is seeing the same background. The child who is well organized at the level of cortex will be able to pass all of these tests unless there is a pathological deterrent to his performance.

We now move on to the evaluation of cortical hemispheric dominance. We evaluate this by ascertaining the handedness, footedness and the pre-dominant eye.

We ask the child to do the following: throw a ball, use scissors, trace a circle, diamond and square with pencil or crayons and to pick up various small objects.

We seek from the parents the hand use for: writing, hammering, eating, brushing teeth and picking up small objects.

We ascertain footedness by asking the child to step up onto a chair, to take large steps forward and backward, to step off a step, and to kick a ball. If there is a real question about footedness, we ask the child to remove his shoes and socks and to pick up various small objects with his toes. If we need further evidence, we ask the child to trace a circle and square with the pencil held in the toes. The child will generally choose the dominant foot. If he is ambivalent and cannot make a choice, we have him draw the circle and square with each foot and we find that the most adeptly drawn figures are drawn with the dominant foot.

The concept of the dominant eye has gone through many variations. We know, as common knowledge, that when one looks into a stereoscope that one image is seen better and is maintained longer. We know that when trying to fuse two colors in a stereoscope one color seems more vivid, while the other tends to be moderately suppressed. We know that there is a phenomenon known as retinal rivalry wherein the image from one eye tends to predominate over the other. We know in the cover test that one eye makes a lesser adjustment than does the other. We know that when testing for near-point convergence one eye holds on to the stimulus after the other has broken the fusion. We know that in strabismus one eye is looking at the stimulus and the strabismic eye is not, it is suppressed. These are all indications that in vision we have a pre-dominance of one eye over the other. In 1961 the author wrote:[3]

"Historically, vision and vision in reading have both been subjected to great investigative variations. At the outset the eyes were studied physiologically and peripherally. The investigations centered on the eye and, somewhat later, on the optic nerve. Brilliant strides were made in gathering knowledge of the eye. Another area of investigation was the field of optics. The discovery and the utilization of the laws of refraction, plus new insights into the nature of light, added new dimensions of treating eyes.

"These two schools of investigation and treatment then moved into the more complex area of binocularity and fusion. Now a new and more elusive variable came into play: the brain. No longer could workers in the field be interested in eyes alone; they now had to take into consideration the entire nervous system. Functional neurology was in its infancy, thus further complicating the problem. Out of this arose the fact that the workers in the field *had to change from dealing with the eyes to dealing with vision.*

"All of the old knowledge fell into a new perspective, because, suddenly, eyes were no longer the subject of investigation; but vision as a part of the whole organism became the subject. There now entered the picture an even more complex variable. Since vision as a part of the whole organism was a dynamic and constantly changing human function, human development became the new area of investigation. This ontogenetic investigation was fruitful and its findings were buttressed by the phylogenetic data which were available. We had now progressed from the detailed study of the eye to a wholistic and developmental approach to vision.

---

[3]Delacato, C. H.: *Manual of Instructions, The Delacato Stero-Reader,* Meadville, Pa., Keystone View Co., 1961, pp. 1-3.

"Eyes could no longer be evaluated or treated as separate entities. Evaluation and treatment had to be developmentally oriented and had to be related to the complete organism. Eyes do not function independently. They cannot be evaluated independently, nor can they be treated independently. *Eyes* had now become *vision*. Vision must be evaluated and treated as a part of the total neurological organization of the individual.

"Concurrent with this activity and following Orton, educators and some neurologists began to investigate vision as it related to reading. It was their premise that, although we knew the physiology of the eye, although we knew how to correct refractive errors, and although we knew some of the neural components of fusion, we did not know the function of vision in the reading process. This investigation studied the relationship between the two eyes in the reading process: the cortical representation of these unknown intravisual relationships.

"By this time "dominance" had been put into the literature, meaning *cortical hemispheric dominance,* and the relationships between the two eyes were investigated in terms of a dominant-subdominant relationship.

"The first great error of this investigative activity resulted in having the *sighting eye* termed the *dominant eye.* This was accepted for a short time, but further investigation, primarily by educators, proved this premise erroneous. The concept of dominance and the dominant eye as it related to reading fell into disrepute, because sighting was used synonymously with dominnance. The error was the result of dealing with the eye instead of the hemisphere that it represented. Although there seemed to be some obvious relationship between visual patterns and language patterns, there was no way in which to validate or use the relationship.

"Some investigators faced with this difficulty of validating the eye-brain relationship and the intravisual relationships moved toward the periphery and studied the eye-hand relationship. Although this investigation made very significant contributions to the field, it represented lower neural levels, both ontogenetically and phylogenetically. Eye-hand coordinations are initiated at a subcortical level and are essentially developed at the mid-brain stage of mobility, which takes place at about nine months of age in the normal child. Eye-hand relationships are prerequisite to language development, but the important factor is *which eye* and *which hand* and *what neural level and hemisphere* do they represent.

"What was needed was a *central neuro-visual approach based on the premise that we do not evaluate or train eyes, but that we evaluate and train neuro-visual patterns and that these patterns are developmental in nature; hence, treatment must be based upon a developmental rationale.*

"The Berners' investigation took a new tack. It operated on the premise that perhaps there might be a better way to study the relationship of the two eyes to each other, which was more reliable than was *sighting.* This lack of reliability had led educators to frown on the concept of the dominant eye. The Berner rationale attempted to study the relationship of the eyes to each other in a functional visual situation. This also implied that inferences could be drawn for the cortical factors involved. The Berners evaluated the vision of each eye while both eyes were seeing. They tested monocular function in a binocular visual situation and found a relationship between the two eyes and were able to use this relationship to diagnose, predict, and treat language problems. Because they were dealing with the eye that controlled the binocular visual situation, they called it the *controlling* eye.

"One objective of all of this investigation was to find the implications for reading resulting from the new knowledge of the relationship of vision to reading and the relationship of vision to neural activity. *It can be assumed that eyes do not work independently and that they must be controlled by the brain.* Therefore, it must follow that knowledge relative to the eyes as they form the concept of *vision* must give us knowledge relative to the *brain.* If we add to this knowledge that which we know, working ontogenetically from neural development to visual development, we can set up a visual schema that, in reality, gives us the data on which we can decide what is the dominant hemisphere visually and what we shall call in this manual the "predominant eye." This schema would give us the following criteria for ascertaining the predominant eye.

>   *Predominant Eye*
>   Sighting—1. Far-point *sighting* (binocular)
>   2. Far-point *sighting* (monocular)
>   3. Near-point *sighting* (binocular)
>   4. Near-point *sighting* (monocular)
>   Control—5. *"Controlling Eye"*—far point
>   (Telebinocular®)
>   6. *"Controlling Eye"*—near point
>   (Telebinocular)
>   Function—7. Eye that reads better (function)
>   8. Eye used for writing (function)

"*The predominant eye is evaluated in terms of, and is composed of, sighting, control, and function.*

"*The predominant eye is merely the visual reflection of the dominant cortical hemisphere.*"

Binocular Sighting—Far-Point

Ask the child to point to a target between the examiner and the child. Have the child keep both eyes open. The examiner then sights from the target, to the child's finger, to the child's eye. The eye in a straight line with the target and the finger is the far-point binocular sighting eye.

Another method is to give the child a tube. Ask him to hold it in two hands and sight a far-point target, using the tube as a telescope. The eye to which he brings the tube is the far-point binocular sighting eye.

Monocular Sighting—Far-Point

Hand the child a piece of paper or cardboard 8½ inches by 11, with a ¼ inch diameter hole in the center. Ask the child to hold the paper in two hands at arms length and have him sight a target through the hole. Have him slowly bring the paper back to his face without losing sight of the target. The eye to which the hole is brought is the far-point monocular sighting eye.

Near-Point Sighting

Place a small X on a sheet of paper. Have the child sit at a desk and place the paper with the X at reading distance. Hand the child a three inch tube with a one-half inch diameter. Ask the child to hold the tube in both hands and to sight the X. Have him slowly bring the tube up to his eye without losing sight of the X. The eye to which the tube arrives, while it is being held in both hands, is the near-point sighting eye.

Far-Point Visual Control

Administer the Keystone Visual Survey tests on the Telebinocular. Tests 4½, 5 and 6 are tests of visual efficiency at far-point. Test 4½ is a binocular test of visual efficiency. Test 5 tests the efficiency of the right eye while both eyes are being used, and test 6 tests the efficiency of the left eye while both eyes are being used. The eye which receives the better score (5-right; 6-left) is the controlling eye at far-point.

Near-Point Visual Control

Administer tests 12, 13, and 14 of the Keystone Visual Survey as per above. Test 12 is binocular visual efficiency at near-point, test 13 is right eye efficiency at near-point, and test 14 is left eye visual efficiency at near-point. The eye which makes the better score (13-right; 14-left) is the near-point controlling eye.

Binocular and Monocular Reading Levels

These can be ascertained by administering the Keystone Diagnostic Series. This series presents reading cards of varying difficulty to be read binocularly, then right eyed, then left eyed through the Telebinocular. The binocular reading cards are used for practice and to set a basal reading level. The monocular reading cards result in a score for each eye in terms of both speed and accuracy. The controlling eye should make the higher score. The score of the most efficient eye is usually equal to the score achieved binocularly. The non-controlling eye usually achieves a lower score than does the controlling eye and than do the two eyes working binocularly.

If the Keystone Diagnostic Series is not available, the binocular and monocular reading levels can be ascertained by using a series of graded textbooks and having the child read them both binocularly and monocularly. Gradually increase the difficulty of the materials. Rate the reading performance as compared to the difficulty level of the materials for binocular reading, then for the left eye and then for the right eye. One eye can easily be occluded with a piece of cardboard while the other is being tested.

For those children for whom a more comprehensive indication is desired with the Keystone Diagnostic series not available, administer two forms of the same reading test, one with the left eye optically occluded and the other with the right eye optically occluded. The difference between the scores should be noted. The higher score is made with the more proficient eye. Also note differences in ease of performance, speed and fatigue.

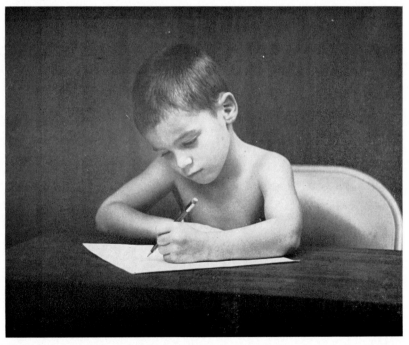

Figure 13. The left handed writer holds his paper at an angle which is opposite to that of the right handed child. Note that the face is slightly rotated toward the right hand, placing the left eye in its most advantageous position for seeing.

Another technique which can be used, if the Keystone materials are not available, is the placing of a reading selection on a card at the mid-line of vision. Ask the child to read the selection while you move it closer and further away from him, very slowly. Watch to see the side toward which the child turns his head. He turns his head so that the predominant eye will be closer to the selection.

Another area of function to be evaluated is that of writing. This should be done with pre-school age children and school-age children. Ask the child to write or to use crayon, if he cannot write. Watch his head position. If his head moves constantly when he writes, either back and forth or from side to side, we know that he is making constant perceptual readjustments. A right-handed child who is using his right eye in a predominant

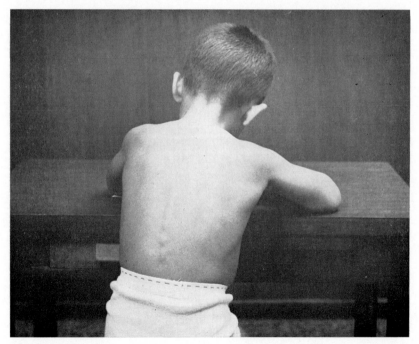

Figure 14. The left handed writer, viewed from the rear. The head is tilted slightly to the right of the spine and the face is rotated slightly toward the right hand, placing the left eye in its most advantageous position for seeing.

role in writing will rotate his head slightly toward the left. This is merely the result of placing the eye in its most advantageous visual axis and can be easily seen by observing the child from the front when he is writing. When observing the child from the rear you will note that the right handed child will tilt the head slightly toward the left of the spine when he is writing correctly.

The left handed child should rotate his face slightly toward his right and his head should be tilted slightly to the right of the spine when he is writing properly (see Figs. 13, 14, 15, and 16).

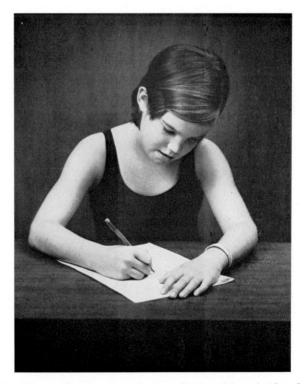

Figure 15. This is the proper paper angle for the right handed writer. The face is rotated slightly toward the left hand and the head is tilted slightly toward the left shoulder, placing the right eye in its most advantageous position for seeing.

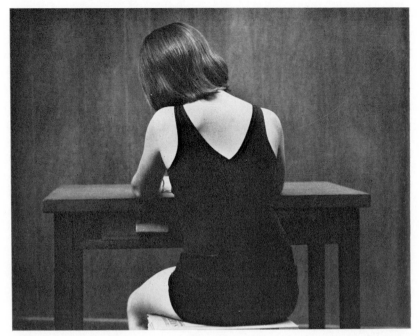

Figure 16. The right handed child, when viewed from the rear, tilts the head to the left of the spine, placing the right eye in its most advantageous position for seeing.

Face rotations or head tilts which do not conform with this pattern are strong indications that the child is using the incorrect eye for predominance of function. Any gross exaggerations of the above patterns are also indications of possible faulty visual function.

We must stress at this point that any functional visual deviation found above should be immediately referred to a visual specialist for further evaluation before initiating treatment.

We have now evaluated the following major factors at the following significant stages of neurological organization.

Cortical Function
    Walking
    Speech
    Vision

DELACATO TEST SUMMARY SHEET[4]

Name:_____ Age:_____ Date:_____

School:_____ Grade:_____

	Right	Left	Mixed
Handedness			
Writing or Crayoning	_____	_____	_____
Throwing	_____	_____	_____
Using Scissors	_____	_____	_____
Brushing Teeth	_____	_____	_____
Eating	_____	_____	_____
Picking Up Small Objects	_____	_____	_____
Footedness			
Stepping Forward	_____	_____	_____
Stepping Back	_____	_____	_____
Stepping onto a Chair	_____	_____	_____
Stepping off a Step	_____	_____	_____
Kicking a Ball	_____	_____	_____
Predominant Eye			
Sighting			
Binocular Sighting at Far-Point	_____	_____	_____
Monocular Sighting at Far-Point	_____	_____	_____
Sighting at Near-Point	_____	_____	_____
Control			
Far-Point Visual Efficiency (Telebinocular)	_____	_____	_____
Near-Point Visual Efficiency (Telebinocular)	_____	_____	_____
Function			
Monocular Reading Level (Keystone Tests of Binocular Skill)	_____	_____	_____
Monocular Reading Level (Informal Reading Inventory)	_____	_____	_____
Writing Position	_____	_____	_____
Earedness (When Necessary)	_____	_____	_____

---

[4]Delacato, C. H.: *Manual of Instructions*, The Delacato Stereo-Reader, Meadville, Pa., Keystone View Co., 1961, p. 11.

Hand and Arm Function
Audition
Affective Behavior

Mid-Brain

Creeping
Vision
Audition
Integrative Behavior

Pons

Crawling
Sleep Pattern
Vision
Audition

Medulla and Spinal Cord

Motility
Mobility

The author feels that these are the minimal criteria which can be used to evaluate the level and quality of neurological organization of a human being. For those who do not meet the criteria we have devised procedures to help them to do so. Only when they meet these criteria can they be considered neurologically well organized. Only when they meet these criteria will they be able to function in the language areas of speech, reading, writing and spelling at a level in keeping with their true capacity.

Chapter 8

TREATMENT PROCEDURES

T HE AUTHOR WISHES to stress that *treatment procedures are synonymous with prevention procedures.* The only difference is that, in treatment, the proper chronological sequence of neurological organization has been disturbed. In prevention, the procedures are generally the same with the function related to neurological organization appearing within the chronology described in Chapter 5.

The author further feels that many of the problems of speech and reading which we are seeing today could have been prevented if the mothers of these children had been cognizant of the significant developmental factors which so greatly influence subsequent neurological organization. Since this chapter deals with treatment procedures, the author will allude only to preventive ramifications. These procedures, if used at the indicated levels of neurological organization, can become the basis of a program for the prevention of speech and reading problems.

Treatment procedures must be related to the central cause of the problem if they are to be successful. They cannot be successful if they are related to the symptoms. We must not, in treatment, fall prey to the common bias of treating symptoms instead of causes.

Let us take the present techniques used by speech therapists as an example. The most important single problem facing the speech therapist is a condition called aphasia. Aphasia is a communication dysfunction resulting from an injury to the brain. It is found in both children and adults. When an injury takes place in the language area of the brain the patient loses his ability to communicate at varying levels; he may lose his gestural ability, speaking ability in many forms, writing ability, reading ability, listening ability or his singing ability. These losses are caused by an injury to the brain—not the eyes in reading, the ears in listening, the hand in writing, and above all not the tongue, lips and larynx in speech. Indeed, if we could miraculously give these aphasic patients new eyes, ears, hands or lips, tongue and larynx, they still would not be able to see, hear, write, read or speak properly. *The cause of the problem is in the brain.* All of the lip exercises, all of the candle blowing exercises and all of the other peripheral techniques generally used by speech therapists are aimed at symptoms and are not aimed at the cause, which is the injured brain.

Speech therapy, if it is to succeed with the aphasic, must be cognizant of the etiology, and treatment must be aimed at the central cause. If the problem lies in the brain, then treatment should deal with the brain. Neurological organization should be used in treating the aphasic.

Reading teachers find themselves in the same dilemma. A problem which is caused by a lack in the nervous system cannot be solved by more or less phonetics, by more or less discipline, by a more or less psychological environment—it must be solved by dealing with the nervous system.

In order to achieve proper neurological organization so that the child can develop those abilities which will enable him to profit from instruction we must first establish a pre-remedial program.

This program is aimed at the central cause of the problem— lack of complete neurological organization. Only after we have solved the central problem will the child be able to profit from instruction. The author has found that the pre-remedial period generally varies from four to twenty weeks to complete. He prefers, during this pre-remedial period, to discontinue all reading or speech instruction unless discontinuation at school places the child in an embarrassing position with his peers. In such instances, the author prefers to have the child continue with reading instruction with as much of the pressure and stress removed from the teaching situation as possible.

The pre-remedial program is initiated at the level of neurological organization indicated by the diagnosis. If the child is completely organized at the level of the spinal cord and the medulla, we begin treatment at the level of pons; if he is completely organized at the level of pons we begin at the level of mid-brain; if he is completely organized at the level of mid-brain we begin at the level of cortex; if he is completely organized at the level of cortex we begin to establish cortical hemispheric dominance. If there is only mild evidence of disorganization at the lower levels we sometimes treat two levels simultaneously.

The only exceptions to the progression of treatment outlined above are those children in the six to eight year age levels who cannot seem to decide on laterality. These are the typical first- and second-grade children who cannot make a choice of handedness, even though they are well beyond the age where children have normally completed the choice. We find that if we go back to the mid-brain level to begin the program that a firmer bi-lateral foundation many times makes for spontaneous progress toward laterality. We feel that this spontaneous progress is the result of a firmer bi-lateral foundation which makes the transition into laterality more facile. The other exception is in the treatment of stuttering. Stutterers profit from a re-enforcement of the bi-lateral functions even if their symptoms of a real lack of neurological organization at this level are mild. The author feels that there is a tendency for stutterers to have made an invalid attempt at cortical organization which tends to mask the mid-brain symptoms.

The child whose neurological organization at the level of the spinal cord and medulla is found lacking is usually severely disabled in terms of mobility. His treatment usually falls within the province of the Rehabilitation Center. The diagnostic and treatment teams of the Rehabilitation Center at Philadelphia have devised two basic methods for enhancing neurological organization at this level.

The first is to allow the child to have every opportunity to use these reflex movements functionally through placing him on the floor for the majority of his waking hours. In the past, restrictions have been placed on these basic movement patterns of disabled children in our efforts to help them to master the cortical function of walking. The error in this approach is that it negates developmental progressions. The expression of these basic patterns is *prerequisite* to the mastery of the more complex patterns of creeping and walking. Since we afford our normal children the opportunity to express these primitive movements, it seems only logical that we should afford the same opportunity for development to our disabled children. Such children should spend the greatest part of their time on the floor.

The second procedure is followed if the child is unable to execute the movements on his own. This procedure involves the passive imposition of the movements upon the body of the child. This passive imposition is aimed at the stimulation of the centers which should be controlling the function but which are not doing so. While one person holds the child's head another moves the body through the undulating fish-like movements typical of this stage. As the child becomes able to express these movements on his own on the floor, we move on to the next level.

The same two procedures are followed where there is a lack of mobility at the level of the pons. For those children who cannot crawl, every opportunity is provided to have them spend as much time as possible on the floor so that they can crawl, if they are able. If the child cannot crawl he is usually disabled.

In addition, homolateral patterning is administered in order to stimulate the responsible brain level. These patterns of movement exactly reproduce the ideal mobility function at this level (see page 72).

For those children who have normal mobility but do not sleep in a proper sleep pattern we have developed two treatment procedures. We first teach the child the proper sleep pattern and explain it to him. We then elicit his cooperation in trying to sleep in the proper position. We further ask the parents to place the child in the proper position when the child is asleep. This is best accomplished by first rotating the child's head in the proper direction. After a few seconds wait, the arms and legs are placed in the proper position.

Second, we find that daily crawling practice with stomach in contact with the floor and using the homolateral pattern is very helpful. We find that a daily five-minute period of homolateral crawling is usually sufficient to establish a proper sleep position in children with normal mobility, in four to eight weeks. For school situations, where space is a problem, we have the child go through the crawling motions on a mat in a stationary position. We find that this patterning without mobility is only slightly less effective than actual crawling with mobility.

Because we all move in our sleep, the position is not maintained throughout the night. In well organized children we find that the movement during sleep tends to be confined to periodic changes from a left sided to a right sided sleep position, with the majority of the time spent in the position which conforms with handedness. If one observes such a sleeping child changing positions from left to right in a homolateral pattern one can readily appreciate the reflex character of the movements. They are smoothly, rhythmically and efficiently executed, even though the child is asleep.

There are environmental variations which affect the sleep positions. Changing the position of the bed in the room or changing the head-foot positions of the bed tends to aid the child in developing the proper sleep pattern. Normal infants who are at the crawling stage should always sleep with the crib sides away from walls, so that environmental factors do not impinge on the development of a proper sleep pattern.

We must be certain that the child who is lacking at this level learns to listen to spoken words. This is the level of the early development of auditory perceptual abilities. The child who is lacking in this development often presents articulation difficulties in his speech or cannot master phonetic elements in his early reading. The procedure is to speak to the child while moving about in his environment. This is first begun with the speaker within the visual field of the child. As soon as the child has mastered the following of the stimulus with the help of vision, the visual cue is deleted. The words are then spoken to the child without having the face of the speaker within the visual field of the child.

The treatment of vision at the level of pons begins in the crawling or sleep pattern. As the child rotates his head toward the left hand he looks at his left hand; as his head rotates toward his right hand, he looks at his right hand. If one observes such a child closely, one notes that he generally looks at the hand with the eye which is in the best position for seeing, the right eye looks at the right hand and the left eye looks at the left hand. Therefore, the actual act of crawling is an excellent method of treating the vision at this level. It is the primary modality for the normal development of vision at this level used by infants.

If further visual treatment is needed at this level it is usually in the area of visual pursuit. We proceed as follows:

1. *Occlude the left eye.* Place a visual stimulus in the form of a small flashlight or pencil in the child's right hand. Have him move his right hand in circular, horizontal, vertical and oblique planes. He will visually pursue the stimulus held in his right hand with his right eye.

2. *Occlude the right eye.* Place a visual stimulus in the child's left hand. Proceed as above. He will visually pursue the stimulus held in his left hand with his left eye.

Three or four one minute periods per day for a period of two to three weeks usually result in bi-ocular vision for a child at this level.

We are helping him to become bi-ocular, which is the visual function at the level of the pons. The important factor of this procedure is that the child must hold the stimulus in his own hand. In the past we have erred in the field of visual training in that we had the parent or therapist hold the target which the child was to pursue visually. This error is easily observed through testing the visual pursuit abilities of children of varying ages. There are many children who visually pursue a moving target crudely and inefficiently, when the target is held by someone other than the child himself. They do so because the placement of the target outside the body and control of the child makes it a cortical function. If we place the target in the child's own hand we find that he can pursue it smoothly and efficiently. He can do so because the hand-eye pursuit is sub-cortically controlled.

Let us digress for a moment to look at this level of vision developmentally. At this level the child should be bi-ocular. At the level of mid-brain he becomes binocular and then at the level of cortex, he finally develops a predominant eye. Many parents have been distressed because they feel that they have allowed an infant to develop fully at each level. Some of these parents have children with faulty neurological organization and cannot understand the reason for it. Such parents feel that they have not biased the child's development toward one side or the other and that they have not interferred with free two-sidedness at lower levels of organization.

Because of a lack of understanding, we have biased our children toward many areas of poor organization. Let us evaluate feeding procedures of today. The infant at the level of the pons developmentally is breast fed in the natural situation. As he suckles from the left breast his right eye is occluded by the breast and his right hand is restricted by the breast feeding position and by the fact that his right arm is at his mother's back. While suckling the left breast he is biased toward total left sided function. At his next feeding he is placed at the right breast. His left eye is occluded by the breast and his left arm is restricted. He is fed from alternate breasts in each successive feeding, one biasing him toward left sidedness and the other toward right sidedness.

When we change this natural situation and bottle-feed the child, we invariably see the right-handed mother hold the baby in her left arm and hold the bottle in her right hand. This is most convenient for the right handed mother, but is detrimental to the infant's neurological organization. Obviously, as she feeds the infant each day she is restricting the use of his right hand and is partially, or wholly, occluding his right eye, forcing the infant toward left sidedness. It would be so simple to revert to the natural alternating right and left sidedness achieved with breast feeding by merely alternating the hand with which the bottle is held and moving the infant from right to left sides on alternate feedings.

At the level of mid-brain, when bilaterality is the developmental objective, feeding again interferes with neurological organization. The mid-brain child of nine months is striving to master complete bi-laterality. His new-found binocularity helps him to locate his food before him and he reaches out for it. He does so bilaterally with his two hands. Too often at this level mothers place a lateralizing influence, such as a spoon, with his food and the end result is teaching a child, who is just becoming properly bilateral, a lateralizing skill. This, when coupled with the many other areas of childhood management which are

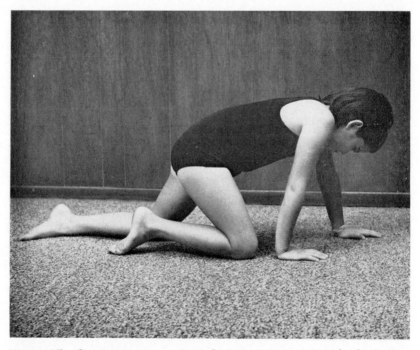

Figure 17. Cross-pattern creeping. It is important to teach the proper hand, arm and head positions and to have the child master the rhythmicity of the movements. Note that the child looks at the forward hand and that the left hand and right knee are moved forward simultaneously.

biasing and restricting in terms of subsequent neurological organization, becomes significant. Children at this level should
never be given eating utensils because utensils require one sidedness and the child is not ready to establish sidedness. Children
at this level should eat with their hands. One can easily observe
that, when children at this level are allowed to eat with their
hands, they universally choose to use both of them. *This should
be encouraged at this age.*

Treatment at the level of mid-brain always begins with mobility. The child is taught to cross-pattern creep properly. He is
taught at the outset how to cross-pattern creep very slowly and
very accurately. The first objective is to have him creep with
the opposite hand and knee striking the floor at the same time.
When this is mastered he is taught to rotate his head slightly
with each step and to look at his forward hand as it strikes the

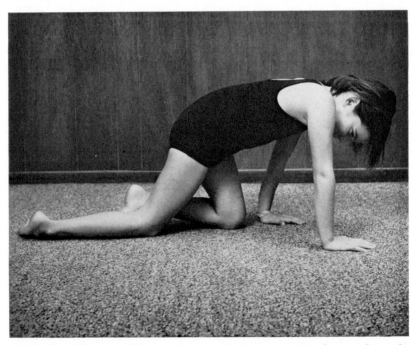

Figure 18. The opposite phase of cross-pattern creeping brings the right
hand and left knee forward with the child again looking at the forward
hand. This movement is performed smoothly and rhythmically.

floor. The result is a simultaneous hand-knee and eye function (see Figs. 17 and 18).

As the cross-pattern creeping becomes smooth and serialized, the following refinements are made:

1. Knees are lifted between each step but feet are dragged along, remaining in constant contact with the floor.
2. Knees are never allowed to cross. They should move forward in two parallel lines.
3. Hands should point forward and palms should be flat on the floor.
4. The head and neck must turn. It is not sufficient to have the eyes rotate from hand to hand.
5. Knees should always be protected, for bruises are apt to develop with continued practice.

The time for mastery of cross-pattern creeping varies very much. Teachers are often discouraged with the difficulty that normal children and adults have in mastering cross-pattern creeping. Our daily practice time recommendations vary from ten minutes per day to one hour per day. We find that in normal school situations three or four fifteen-minute periods per week of cross-pattern creeping is sufficient for the establishment of good cross-pattern skills, for up to 90 per cent of the student body. Schools which have special education, remedial reading and classes for the brain injured need more time per week. We also find practically no resistance on the part of the children to do cross-pattern creeping. This is especially true if they practice in group situations.

Visual development at this level is greatly enhanced by cross-pattern creeping. As the child creeps in cross-pattern he turns his head and looks at his forward hand. This constantly changing head and neck position provides constantly changing sensory-motor cues to the eyes. In short, these added cues help the eyes to learn where they are looking. This extra-sensory motor stimulation, especially from the neck, helps the eyes learn where they are looking and, indeed, helps them to learn at the early stages of visual development what they are looking at. This stim

ulation is a basic prerequisite to the development of the yoking
of the two eyes so that they begin to function in concert.

Further visual training at this level consists of visual pursuit
of a moving target with both eyes simultaneously. The movements should be circular, horizontal, vertical and oblique and
they should begin with the child holding the moving target in
his own hands. The hands are alternated for those children who
have no preferred hand. The treatment is binocular and self-
directed. As complete yoking is established and as the pursuit
is mastered into a smooth and efficient pattern the target is
placed in the hand of someone other than the child. The child
must now learn to follow the target while it is being directed by
someone else.

The person who moves the target should make the motions
large enough so that the child has to move his head to keep the
target in view. The therapy has moved from the sub-cortical
hand-eye relationships to early cortical visual function when this
is mastered. Three or four one-minute periods per day are usually sufficient to strengthen fragile binocularity in approximately
one month's time. Severe lacks of binocularity, such as exists in
the strabismic, will require more time each day over a two- or
three-month period.

Music and tonal discrimination and memory play a part in
the treatment at the mid-brain level. Children who are disorganized at this level should have ample opportunity to listen
to music. We find that primitive folk-type melodies are the most
effective. We have children at this level listen to such songs
for ten-minute periods three or four times per week. We find
that instrumental records are not as effective as vocal records in
helping to develop the early tonal memory (which is probably
a form of conditioning) and auditory discrimination at this level.

Much talking and some reading aloud by an adult are helpful
to children at this level. When reading aloud, have the child
look away from the reader. It is sometimes helpful to give the
child paper and crayons and to allow him to draw while he is
listening. This is the area in which the use of television is helpful. Television sound should be reduced slowly till it is barely

audible while the child watches a clear picture. Another procedure is to have the sound loud and clear while the picture is
somewhat dark or hazy. Games requiring sounds and memory
of sounds are also helpful at this level.

A great majority of children who present articulation problems in speech, delayed speech, or are unable to master phonetic
elements in reading, are generally poorly organized in this area
and profit from these activities. Children who are disorganized
at this level should be taught to play games using large balls
which require two hands. They should be encouraged to play
foot games requiring the use of both feet.

The overall evaluation of the success of the therapy at the
level of the mid-brain is the complete mastery of bilateral activity. This includes bimanual, bipedal, binaural and binocular
functions. When mastered, they can be performed in a very
smooth and synergistic fashion.

A phenomenon which one often sees, when the mid-brain level
is mastered, takes place with hyperactive children. They tend
to become calmer and more attentive and their distractibility decreases significantly. This is probably the result of increased integrative ability which, in many areas of function, is the province
of the mid-brain.

Treatment at the cortical level begins with the mastery of
cross-pattern walking. The child is taught to step off with either
foot. He is taught to point at that foot with his opposite hand.
He then steps with the other foot and again points to it with
the opposite hand. When he steps with his left foot he points
with his right hand, when he steps with his right foot he points
with his left hand. The process of pointing to the opposite foot
is made easier and more natural when the upper body is turned
slightly from the waist. As the child points to the opposite foot
his head and body turn toward the foot to which he is pointing.

The child is then taught to look at the forward hand as he uses
it to point to the opposite foot. As the hand comes toward the
opposite foot it is in the periphery of the visual field. It moves
from the periphery toward the center of the visual field until the
foot strikes the floor. At this point the hand points at the foot

and the child visually fixates the hand macularly. Here again we repeat the hand-eye-foot pattern of cross-pattern creeping. The only difference is that the child is upright (see Figs. 11 and 12).

The reader will note that cross-pattern walking as described is merely the exaggeration of what we all know as normal walking. We have found that it is not as difficult to master as is cross-pattern creeping. This is no doubt the result of earlier mastery of cross-pattern creeping prior to the initiation of cross-pattern walking. As cross-pattern walking is being mastered, the following refinements are made:

1. Practice should be done in bare feet.
2. Legs must not cross. They must move forward in parallel lines.
3. Child should toe out slightly.
4. Speed of walking should be varied during practice sessions.
5. The observer must make certain that the child rotates his head, neck and eyes toward the forward hand with each step.
6. With each step have the child visually fixate the forward hand while maintaining visual consciousness of the foot below the hand.

For those children who have difficulty in mastering smooth cross-pattern walking we recommend that they practice at a slow trot or that they practice on an incline or a hill. We find that the change in gravitational force tends to modify the movement synergy.

We usually prescribe daily ten-minute periods of cross-pattern walking during the pre-remedial period. This is usually easily accomplished at home. We have found it very satisfactory to include this practice in the physical education program of schools. We have also found that there is little resistance to this activity on the part of school children or college students.

Auditory training at this stage includes much discussion, primarily at a peer group level. The child at this level learns many of the nuances of spoken language from his contemporaries

Children with delayed speech or with articulation problems are often ridiculed by their peers. The most significant language function at this level is the appearance of the developmental stutter. As the child begins to move toward laterality, both hemispheres are being used in most acts. At that point where the two hemispheres are balanced in the control of the functions a stutter or an indecision appears. The stutter continues until one hemisphere becomes somewhat dominant for that set of acts. This is usually a very short time in well organized children, lasting for a few days. In poorly organized children the stutter may persist for weeks. If it persists beyond that the child is known as a stutterer.

If one evaluates a developmental stutterer, one finds that the acts wherein he is indecisive are many. He, therefore, does not only stutter in his speech, he stutters in his vision, his mobility and in his audition. Since speech is the most conscious and the most complex act, it is the area in which the stutter is most obvious.

Stuttering children who enjoy music, or who listen to a more than average amount of music, should begin a gradual process of deletion of music from the environment. It is replaced by story-telling records, choral speaking, rhythmic activity and poetry. The child at this level is becoming ready to begin to establish cortical hemispheric dominance. When he does so, music is relegated to a sub-dominant role.

This is the stage of large muscle development and coordination. Any form of play activity which requires the use of large muscle groups is very helpful. The play should be of the free-play type and should give the child many varied functional experiences upon which he can begin to make early and tentative choices of sidedness.

Visual training no longer requires visual pursuit. The child at the level of cortex is refining the simultaneous use of his two eyes and is learning to fuse the two perceptions arriving at the visual areas of the cortex. He is developing stereopsis. Visual training deals with the child's adjustment to his relationship in space and that of the world about him, if he is properly organized up to this level. His basic adjustments are to variations in distance. The child now learns to see in the third dimension. He learns from the occulo-motor adjustments which he must make; he learns through a building of apperceptions; he learns through applying cultural knowledge to his perceptions and he learns through trial and error about his own position in space and that of the objects which he sees in space.

Most of the learning can be achieved through normal play activity. Games which deal with balls, varying distances and discrimination of targets at far- and near-points, are helpful. These activities must depend, of course, upon the proper development of binocularity which is prerequisite to visual success at this level. This is the stage when many visual problems develop. It is a stage of dynamic maturity of the whole visual process.

Training procedures depend on much running, jumping, and general activity on the part of the child. For those cases who are very poor at this level, push-ups are helpful. The child holds a visual target in his hand at arms length. While looking at the target he slowly brings it closer to his face. In addition, practice in having him look at targets at varying distances in his environment on command is also helpful. This is easily accomplished by parents at home or in a school situation by asking the child to look at objects placed at varying visual distances about the room. As the teacher names the object, the children look at it. We have found this to be a popular classroom game.

As the child masters stereopsis and becomes able to place himself and his visual world in the proper spatial relationships, he becomes ready to move on to the next visual adjustment required at the level of cortex. He must learn to become a gradually increasing near-point human being in visual terms. This requires the gradual development of tolerance to stress required to use the eyes at near-point. The child's world up to this point has been a far-point world, which is a fairly comfortable world in visual terms. As he moves closer to reading he must develop the ability to sustain near-point vision and he must become able to do so without undue stress or fatigue.

Bringing a child to near-point merely requires giving him near-point tasks, such as model building, crayoning, or writing. Those children who cannot accept the stress at this juncture often refuse to do them. If they are being taught to read, they either refuse to do so, or dislike reading. At this juncture, the visual specialist is a strong ally. Many children develop severe myopia because they cannot make this visual adjustment. Many children develop problems of stress, hyperactivity and in some instances, emotional problems when called upon to make this adjustment. The author feels that constant visual evaluations must be made by a visual specialist as the child is being brought from a far-point to a near-point world.

As the preremedial period encompasses these cortical functions, the child should be scheduled for visual evaluations to ascertain the adjustments which he is making to a near-point world in the form of beginning reading and writing.

We must digress for a moment to view a treatment area which has afforded results with no apparent rationale. Getman[1] and Kephart[2] and the members of the Optometric Extension Program report significant success in developing vision with brain injured and normal children, using as the primary treatment modality— the trampoline.

Those who use the trampoline attribute their results in better visual performance and better mobility to somewhat peripheral factors. They feel that the trampoline improves balance, visual accommodation, etc. with no complete rationale as to its use or the reason why it apparently succeeds in a number of cases and in a number of areas.

With the publication of the *Treatment and Prevention of Reading Problems* in 1959 the author became the recipient of a number of case histories with impressive results, through the use of the trampoline. The author was asked to explain these results which were not the result of neurological organization but which were, instead, the result of the peripheral factors mentioned by those who used the trampoline.

---

[1]Getman, G. N.: How to Develop Your Child's Intelligence, Pub. by the Auth, Luverne, Minn., 1959.
[2]Kephart, N.: *The Slow Learner in The Classroom*, Columbus, Ohio, Charles E. Merrill Co., 1960.

We decided to investigate the use of the trampoline to see whether it was a repudiation of the concepts of neurological organization. We found that the trampoline was invented by a French Neurologist who named it the Trampolino. He used it to treat brain injured children, with some success.

One cannot ascertain any relationship to the nervous system if one watches children jumping on a trampoline. We viewed twenty normal children on the trampoline but saw nothing to help in ascertaining any relationships. We then set up a camera and took a series of still pictures of children jumping on a trampoline. The results were most revealing and explained the effectiveness of the trampoline.

We move through neurological organization in a set pattern from lower levels to higher levels. This, in essence, is a horizontal treatment procedure taking one step at a time and going sequentially from lower to higher levels of organization.

We found that when we placed a child on a trampoline *we negated this horizontal and logical developmental pattern but that, in essence, the whole pattern of neurological organization was crudely recreated with each jump.*

As the child leaves the gravitational pull to which he is accustomed, by jumping on the trampoline, the springing action exerts a greater force than does the gravitational pull to which the child is accustomed, and as a result, he goes through very interesting changes in neurological organization. He is going from higher levels of organization, as he starts, and goes to lower levels as the jump progresses, returning to the cortical level when he returns to his original gravitational state. As he jumps, various levels of the nervous system become dominant as he progresses from the beginning of the jump to the apex and back to the beginning of the next jump (see Figs. 19 to 25).[3]

At the height of the jump and at any time during the ensuing free fall all parts of the body are moving at the same speed due to the force of gravity. Since all parts of the body are moving at the same rate there is an experience of weightlessness. As

---

[3]Fay, T.: The Thumb as A Clinical Aid in Diagnostic Screening of Paralysis, *J. A. M. A., 155:*729-732, June, 1954.

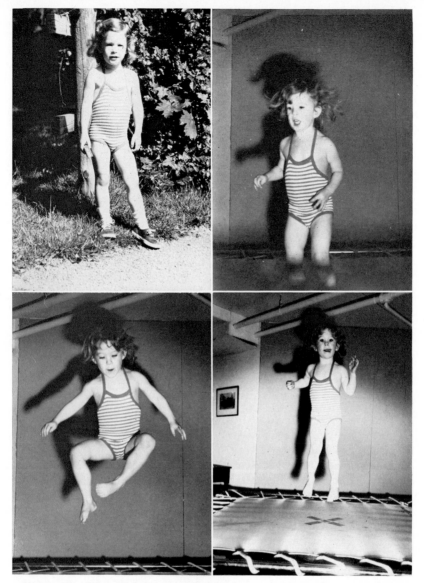

Figure 19. Normal three year old child prior to using the trampoline.
Figure 20. Note the great disorganization. Note the bilateral cortical thumbs and the mildly athetoid facial features.
Figure 21. Thumbs are in a more normal cortical position. Facial features are typical of the mid-brain injured (athetoid), Babinsky is at its height. Note the toes are in a perfect Babinsky, which in a child of this age would normally be considered an indication of pathology. Vision is clearly binocular.
Figure 22. As the child leaves the pad notice the thumbs. Both of them are in the cortical thumb position found in children who are injured at the level of cortex. Note the mask-like features typical of the mid-brain injured (athetoid). The level of Pons is operative, note the tonic-neck position of the head and arms. This is not usually present in the waking state after sixteen weeks of life. Note the haziness of the binocularity.

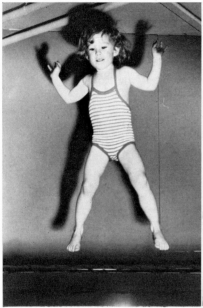

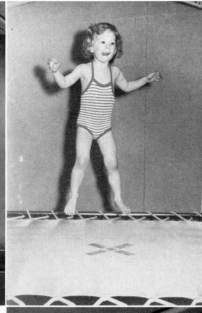

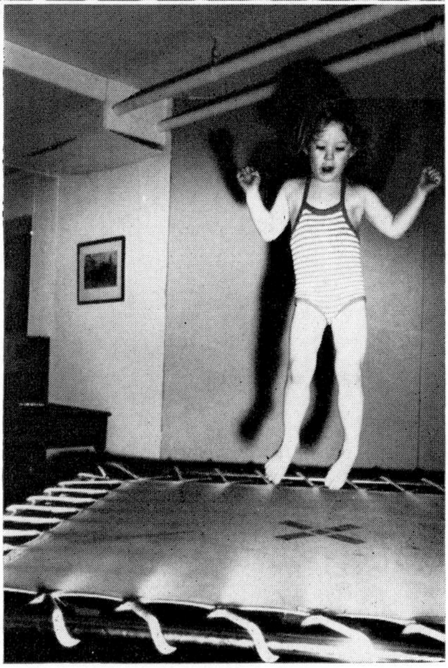

Figure 23. At the apex of the jump the child appears truly bilateral. Note the binocularity of vision and the seeming state of rest in which the body is suspended.

Figure 24. The body has become more bilateral. There is only one cortical thumb, the other is normal. The facial features are still somewhat athetotic. Vision is more binocular.

Figure 25. Note the thumbs in the palms typical of the cortically injured child. The body is in a bilateral attitude typical of the intact mid-brain. Note the Babinsky reflex (withdrawal of the feet), which is normal up to the age of two and is pathological reflex after that age. Note that binocularity is present here.

soon as contact is made with the trampoline the retarding force is transmitted into the rest of the body. This force reaches a maximum at the bottom of the trampoline motion, at which time deceleration is greatest. As the child again leaves the trampoline he again experiences weightlessness. The variation from weightlessness to strong deceleration provides a dynamic gravitational environment rarely experienced by children. It results in a new and constantly changing stimulation and reaction pattern to be experienced by the entire nervous system.

The vertical stimulation of the nervous system stimulates the consecutive neural levels toward greater neurological organization. Because of its bilateral nature it cannot do so at the level of hemispheric dominance. The trampoline can be helpful for those children who are poorly organized at the level of midbrain and early cortex *only*. Children who are disorganized below those levels could not use the trampoline because of their disability, and those who have not developed hemispheric dominance would not profit from its use, for it is completely bilateral in function.

The program of neurological organization outlined in this book goes vertically from the lowest level to the highest level in consecutive developmental levels, i.e., medulla, pons, mid-brain, cortex, and then hemispheric dominance. As each stage is mastered, we go on to the next stage, as do all normal children. The trampoline stimulates each area with each jump. As the child leaves the trampoline (his gravitational base) his cortex loses its dominance in controlling function. He finds it difficult to consciously change his patterns of movement while in the air. When he returns to the trampoline he again functions cortically. The same phenomenon can be seen in diving. Excellent divers take a long time just standing on the diving board before an intricate dive, to go over the various movements required to complete the dive consciously. When they leave the diving board they cannot cortically control their movements because the cortex loses much of its ability to dominate when the diver loses his familiar gravitational environment. Excellent divers spend the pause before the dive, going over the details of the dive cortically (consciously), because once the dive starts they cannot change the course of the dive as they wish they could. They are, in essence, "programming" the nervous system before starting the dive.

All of the procedures for the establishment of cortical hemispheric dominance must be followed simultaneously. Each of the areas needs the re-enforcement of the others. The author wishes to stress the fact that we are not training a foot, an eye or a hand, but that we are in fact retraining a hemisphere of the brain. The retraining of one area alone cannot result in the establishment of hemispheric dominance.

Hemispheric dominance is established through the increasingly selective, receptive and expressive function of one side of the body. Children who are unable to become completely one-sided need much environmental help to aid in the establishment of dominance. One-sidedness, which in turn reflects hemispheric dominance, is prerequisite to reading and complete speech, hence, training at this level takes place within the pre-remedial period. One-sidedness means that one hand becomes the skilled hand, one foot becomes the skilled foot and one eye becomes the predominant eye. They must all be on the same side.

Left sided children have the greatest difficulty at this level because they live in a right handed world. Their environments are geared to the convenience of right handed people who predominate numerically by a 9 to 1 ratio. As a result, the dominance of the left sided ten per cent of our population is constantly being challenged by the environment instead of being re-enforced by the environment.

Right sided children who represent the great numerical majority of the population have similar difficulties, in that there are cultural influences which tend to confuse them. If we return to our earlier example of cultural confusion, that of feeding and eating practices, we find that there are many cultural biases which tend to challenge the complete development of dominance. The placement of eating utensils is most confusing. Since some are placed on the right and some on the left, the child's laterality is being challenged instead of being re-enforced every time he eats. All utensils and glasses should be placed at the left for left handed children and they should all be placed at the right for right handed children. This is true of all children from the ages of four through eight and is especially true of children who are having difficulty in establishing complete laterality.

The first treatment procedure at this level is to delete tonality from the child's environment as much as is possible. This is somewhat traumatic to brain injured children, to children with even slight aphasia and to stutterers. It is *especially* important that *these* children not have tonality. The deletion of tonality from the environment is traumatic to them for the same reason that they have the communication problem—they have not established complete cortical hemispheric dominance. The deletion of tonality includes completely stopping the listening to music in all forms. Children should not be allowed to attend music classes or music lessons at school or at home. The deletion of music should continue until hemispheric dominance is established.

The viewing of television may be allowed if the sound is turned down so that it is barely audible and if the television has a bright, clear picture.

The deletion of tonality at times causes a form of sound starvation. The child for a period of two or three weeks becomes noisy in many of his activities. He tends to hum more than he did, to bang objects together, to whistle, to pound his feet as he walks and to tap things with his fingers or with small objects, all in an effort to produce sounds to which he can listen. As this starvation period ends there ensues a quieter behavior pattern. This change toward greater quiet is most striking with the hyperactive child for he becomes calmer and less hyperactive as the dominant-subdominant tonal relationships are established. This has been seen by others in the field of brain injury,[4] in that such children tend to become more able to pay attention and to learn in an unstimulated environment.

---

[4]Cruikshank, W., Bentzen, F., Ratzeburg, F., and Tannhauser, M.: *A Teaching Method for Brain-Injured and Hyperactive Children*, Syracuse Univ. Press, 1961, pp. 1-576.

For a small minority of about 3 to 5 per cent who arrive at this stage of neurological organization attempting to make both hemispheres skilled hemispheres in terms of sound, the opposite is true. This small group is composed of monotones. They neither enjoy music nor can they carry a tune. They must be returned to the mid-brain level of tonality and must be taught how to discriminate tones and how to carry a tune. Following their mastery of these aspects of tonality they must be treated as above and music must be deleted from the environment. It is interesting to note that the level of intelligence of this small percentage runs significantly higher than that of the too tonal group.

During the time that music is added to the environment of this small group there will be noted a greater tendency toward hyperactivity and inattention. As we watch such children listen to music we note a greater calmness and growing enjoyment during the actual process of listening. Immediately after they have listened to the music, however, there is a greater tendency toward hyperactivity. After the tonality is mastered and as we proceed to delete it from the environment, the greater calm and the cessation of hyperactivity, as described above, ensues.

Concurrently, the sleep pattern of the child, in a pattern consistent with the sidedness which is being trained, must be stressed. It should be developed completely by this stage of treatment, but, if it is not, a greater effort on the part of the parents is to be made to have the child's sleep pattern conform with his sidedness.

Footedness is a somewhat unpredictable area of treatment. It is difficult to prognosticate the mastery of footedness efficiently. This is probably the result of the many cultural influences upon footedness and of the increasingly less complex function required of feet. The mastery of footedness begins with teaching the child to use the dominant foot for activities requiring the use of the feet. This includes kicking, stepping off to walk or to run, balancing and the hurdling of obstacles. There are many playground games which can be used to reenforce or to train footedness.

If there is difficulty in the establishment of a dominant foot, greater sensory stimulation of the foot is helpful. We achieve this by having the child walk about the house wearing a shoe on his sub-dominant foot and without a shoe or stocking on the foot being trained for dominance. Footedness can also be trained by having the child practice picking up small objects with the training foot while barefooted and also while wearing stockings. In extreme cases, we have the child trace sandpaper letters and rough objects with his foot, trying to recognize them without looking at them. In the most extreme cases, we have the child hold a pencil in his toes and first learn to copy simple figures, being sure to go from left to right. This is followed by having him learn to write the alphabet and the numbers from one to ten with his dominant foot in these rare, very extreme cases.

The establishment of a dominant hand is made easier if the hand is first taught early perceptual skills. For those cases where great difficulty is encountered, basic training in feeling surfaces and in becoming conscious of movement are helpful. Tracing of sandpaper pictures or letters,[5] copying figures on a large blackboard,[6] and using large crayons are helpful.

Games requiring the use of one hand as the skilled hand and the other as the assistive hand are helpful. Bilateral activity, such as playing the piano, playing drums, making models, two handed games should all be discouraged at this stage.

The child should be taught to master the following skills with what will become the dominant hand: *throwing, cutting, using scissors, handling of tools, brushing teeth, combing hair, reach-- ing, picking up small objects, gesturing and finally writing.*

The retraining of writing should be the last manual skill retrained. As the other manual skills are mastered the child should be taught to write letters and numbers at a standing blackboard. He should use large letters. They should be at least 6 inches high at the outset. He should gradually diminish the size of the

---

[5]Rambusch, N.: *Learning How to Learn,* Baltimore, Md., Helicon Press, 1962, pp. 1-180.
[6]Kephart, N.: *The Slow Learner in the Classroom,* Columbus, Ohio, Charles E. Merrill, 1960, pp. 1-292.

letters until they are well formed at a height of 2 inches. The child is then moved on to practice his writing with paper and pencil. He should then be encouraged to gradually diminish the size of his writing.

The author wishes to caution the reader at this point relative to possible language interference when the writing hand is changed. On rare occasions language flow decreases, or a stutter appears as a result of changing handedness. If this happens, a complete evaluation of the mastery and retention of sub-cortical organization should be made. If it is not complete, or if it has not been retained, it should be completed. If the sub-cortical organization is complete, an evaluation should be made of those other activities which are being followed in attempting to establish hemispheric dominance. Without a complete program, stuttering may appear.

It is an error to change only the hand in attempting to establish hemispheric dominance. This quite often causes stuttering. Before changing handedness, sub-cortical organization must be complete. While changing handedness, footedness must be changed, sleep pattern must be followed, tonality must be deleted, and the predominant eye must be established.

If these other functions of cortical dominance are not re-enforced, the changing of the hand alone adds to the child's confusion and stuttering may develop. The reason is simple. We are not dealing with hands, eyes and feet, but we are instead dealing with cortical hemispheric dominance. We are not attempting to change the hand, foot and eye, but we are attempting to reorganize that part of the nervous system which controls the hand, foot and eye.

The establishment of a predominant eye must begin at far-point. Children should be taught to wink the subdominant eye and to look at far-point monocularly. They should be taught to sight with the predominant eye at far-point both binocularly and monocularly. Games requiring telescopes or looking through apertures are excellent aids in having the child make proper sighting choices at far-point. Microscopes, or near-point games requiring sighting, help to establish proper sighting at near-point.

We next help the child to develop an eye which predominates in the binocular visual act. The author has labeled this eye the *Predominant Eye*. See page 94.

The establishment of a predominant eye in the visual pattern is a slow but consistent process in normal development. It begins with the mastery of binocularity. The predominant eye is usually established by the age of eight. Training a predominant eye requires the training of a single eye in perceptual skills while not threatening the integrity of the child's binocularity. We have the following methods for the training of the predominant eye. They are placed in order from the least desirable to the most desirable.

1. *Direct occlusion of the Eye.*
2. *Optical occlusion of the Eye.*
3. *Filtering out the Visual Image.*
4. *Stereo-Reader.*

1. Direct occlusion of the eye is achieved by placing an opaque patch directly over the eye. The author originally subscribed to occlusion of the sub-dominant eye for the development of a predominant eye. Subsequent investigation has led the author to conclude that occlusion is not the most effective method of retraining. Its basic weakness is that, with those children who have fragile binocularity, occlusion tends to make the binocular function weaker. This is the result of totally eliminating the vision from the non-trained eye. It reduces the normally binocular reading situation to a totally monocular situation.

2. Optical occlusion of the eye is achieved through placing a mottled lens over the non-training eye, or through making opaque one lens of a non-prescription pair of glasses. The point of occlusion moves from no sight in direct occlusion to about 1 inch away from the eye in optical occlusion. Optical occlusion has the added advantage over direct occlusion that the eye sees light, where it does not even see light in direct occlusion. The weakness of optical occlusion lies in the fact that the point of occlusion is only 1 inch from the eye, making the functional visual situation basically monocular. Although the eye can see light, it cannot see anything else and it is not perceiving the stimulus.

3. Filtration of the visual image so that it is not seen by the non-training eye can be achieved by passing light through two lenses, which set the light vibrating in opposite directions. For example, if we placed a lens over the non-training eye which was polarized from top to bottom, it would allow only light which was vibrating vertically to come through the lens. If we placed a plate of glass over the book to be read, which was polarized from right to left, the light coming through the glass would vibrate from left to right. As it met the lens it would be extinguished, for the lens would allow only light which was vibrating vertically to pass through. As a result, the eye wearing the lens would not be able to see anything behind the glass plate. This same phenomenon can be achieved with various combinations of colored filters, one color filter worn over the eye vibrating the light in one direction and another color filter placed over the reading material vibrating the light in an antagonistic direction. The result is the occlusion of the reading material from the eye at the point of prime contact, which is at the second filter from the eye or the filter which is placed on the book. This method moves the point of occlusion out into space. This point exists *at* the book. This is an improvement over the other two methods, since it more closely resembles a binocular visual act. The fact remains, however, that the visual image going to the brain is a one-sided image. The training eye is perceiving the stimulus but the other eye is receiving a distorted image and that distorted image is being transmitted to the brain. What was needed was a training procedure which maintained binocularity or more ideally re-enforced binocularity while training a predominant eye perceptually.

As can be seen from the above, what was needed was a training procedure which trained the predominant eye in perceptual and reading skills, while not inhibiting the function of the non-training eye. The ideal situation would be to be able to train the predominant eye perceptually while the other eye was seeing. This requires monocular training in a binocular visual situation.

The author devised the Stereo-Reader, which is such a training device.[7] See Figure 26.

⟫→

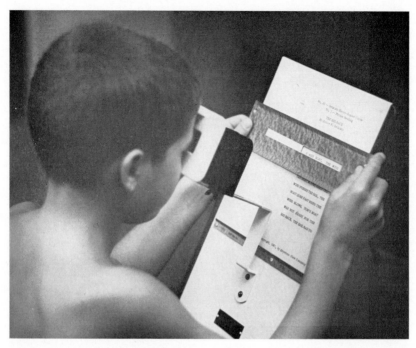

Figure 26. The Stereo-Reader places the material directly in front of the eye which is being trained. Because of the consistent background the other eye is seeing while the training eye is perceiving. This child is training the right eye. (Courtesy Keystone View Co., Meadville, Pa.)

The Stereo-Reader consists of a stereoptic eyepiece facing a reading surface upon which visual training materials and reading materials can be placed. They can be placed so that they can be seen with only one eye at a time. The stereoscopic effect coupled with the common background for both eyes gives the reader the illusion that he is seeing the training materials with both eyes. This is a form of visual projection such as is found in chiroscopic drawing. A reading guide is placed over the training materials which enhances the illusion because its construction and color blend with the visual figure-ground structure. The reading guide can be adjusted to be used for left or right sided training.[8]

[7]Manufactured and distributed by the Keystone View Company, Meadville, Pennsylvania.

➤

The training materials include 10 Visual Motor, 6 Word Families, 5 Visual Discrimination, 16 Phrase Reading, 103 Reading for Interest, and 12 Speed Reading exercise cards.

The Stereo-Reader achieves the objectives listed above in that it does not occlude the eye, it merely places the materials in such a position that the non-training eye cannot see it, although it sees the same background. *It is, in essence, training one eye to perceive while both eyes are seeing.* This provides no threat to binocularity; in fact, it re-enforces binocularity because, via visual projection, the child feels that he is seeing the training materials with both eyes, although he really can see them only with the eye which is being trained.

For those extreme cases of poor binocularity, or for those cases which need simultaneous binocular training and the development of the pre-dominant eye, The Stereo-Reader is modified so that binocularity can be controlled and measured. A horizontal line drawn across the yellow portion of the reading guide one-third of the distance up from the bottom of the yellow section provides such a control. Using the line as a binocular control, the child is asked to underline everything read with a black line. If the *line* disappears, we know he is suppressing the non-training eye. If the *writing* disappears, we know he is suppressing the training eye. As long as he sees the training material *underlined* we know that he is using both eyes and we know that only the training eye is being trained to perceive. We have with this modification achieved the antithesis to occlusion in that we have a controlled binocular visual situation in which only one eye is being trained (see Fig. 26).

We have found using the Stereo-Reader for twenty minutes per day to be of significant value in establishing a predominant eye. We also find that its use in classroom, clinic or home training situations is easily supervised because its use does not require specialized personnel after the original orientation to the instrument.

---

[8]Delacato, C. H.: *Manual for Delacato Stereo-Reader*, Meadville, Pa., Keystone View Co., 1961, pp. 1-23.

We use the Stereo-Reader developmentally for those first- and second-grade children who are in the process of developing a predominant eye. It has been used extensively in normal classrooms as an aid in furthering this development for children who have no significant problems in language, but who are having some mild difficulty in establishing a predominant eye. We find that four daily ten-minute periods per week of using the Stereo-Reader makes a significant difference in such cases.

The position in which the child holds his head is very important to the development of a predominant eye, both developmentally and in treatment. The right handed child should be taught to rotate his head slightly toward the left and to tilt it slightly toward the left when writing. This places the predominant eye in the most advantageous axis for seeing. The left handed child should be taught to rotate the head slightly toward his right and to tilt his head slightly toward the right when writing. This places the left eye at the most advantageous axis for seeing (see Figs. 13 to 16).

The child should be taught to hold his paper correctly. He should hold the paper tilted at a 45 degree angle and the angle should conform with his sidedness.

The proper head and face position, coupled with the proper paper position, is very difficult to achieve at the beginning of treatment. The child usually turns his body in the chair or writes up or down hill. It is important that the process begin slowly with the mastery of the head positions. As this is mastered, teach the child how to sit squarely at a desk. Then place strips of adhesive tape on his desk as outlines for his paper. They should be placed at an angle which is 5 degrees closer to the correct 45 degree angle, shown in Figures 13 and 15. As the child masters this angle, the adhesive strips are moved to an angle which is an added 5 degrees closer to the ideal. This continues until the child achieves the correct angle. Care must be taken throughout that the head rotation and tilt remain in the proper position and that the child continues to sit with his body facing the desk properly.

The child should be taught the proper distance for near-point work. Eyes which are too close to the page increase the visual stress on the child and, eyes which are too far away distort the fixation point. The easiest method for ascertaining the proper distance and for teaching it to the child is to have the child make a fist. The distance between his elbow and first knuckle on the closed hand is the proper distance. He can easily measure this by placing his elbow on the paper and having his forearm and clenched fist make up the distance between the paper and the child's eyes. Having set the distance, the child can begin to read or write. If he moves, he can easily place his elbow on the paper and his clenched fist at his eye to reset the proper distance.[9]

The pre-remedial program should be followed for from four to six weeks. At that time a re-evaluation of the child's neurological organization should be made. As the child masters the lower levels of organization he should be moved on to the next higher levels.

The author has experienced considerable success in teaching these procedures to parents and having them supervise the program in their homes. A monthly re-evaluation is advisable during the pre-remedial period.

School programs which are remedial, preventive or developmental in nature are relatively easily supervised by the classroom teacher with the help of the physical education department and the school nurse. Re-evaluations at the school level are easily accomplished if these personnel use a team approach.

The teaching of either speech or reading should follow this general sequence:

Learning by Wholes

The child should be introduced to words conceptually. They should arise from his experience. Children can learn to say or to read whole words if the word has real meaning for them. As the child begins to master whole words at a speech or reading level, we move on to a slightly more detailed level of teaching.

---

[9]Harmon, D. B.: Notes on a Dynamic Theory of Vision, Pub. by the author, Austin, Texas, 1958.

Contextual Learning

The child is helped to recognize words by learning about their relationships to other words and to the sense of the sentence. Such word relationship cues are helpful in the greater mastery of word attack, in increasing comprehension and, more importantly, in increasing the mastery of word meanings.

Structural Analysis

In speech, this involves the global study of the saying of a word and a consciousness of the small meaningful word components which make up our words. In reading, the emphasis is placed on breaking up large words into their smaller components. This is also the time to teach configurational, or outline, cues to word analysis. Children who have had difficulty with reading need much practice in learning to observe configurational variations. They tend to be able to learn large words with varied configurations but have great difficulty mastering small words because of the lack of configurational variations in small words.

Phonetic Analysis

The next step is to present to the child the phonetic elements of speech and reading. This should always start with skills—the consonants. As the consonants are being mastered, the vowel sounds are introduced. This should be done slowly and with a minimum of emphasis on the techniques involved. The study of phonetics should be an aid to reading. It should not be mastered as a body of knowledge, but as a set of skills used as aids in mastering the process of speech or reading.

Repeat the Process

As the child moves from conceptual wholes to smaller components certain masteries occur. When the child reaches a plateau, begin the whole process again.

The general technique, therefore, goes from learning by wholes to contextual learning, to structural analysis, to phonetic analysis back to learning by wholes and the repetition of the process.

Plateaus in speech progress are readily observed and the astute therapist immediately returns to conceptual learning when they appear.

As reading is mastered, the cycle from whole word learning to phonetic analysis becomes larger and longer. During this early period of reading instruction the size of the materials read should be as large as possible, making the visual stress required as minimal as possible.

All verbal and experiential discussion of early reading should be done aloud. Oral reading, however, should always be preceded by silent reading, and *oral reading should always be done in whispers.*

Reading instruction should always be accompanied with writing instruction dealing with the same words. The writing of the words tends to re-enforce the reading mastery and also, when done properly, re-enforces the establishment of cortical hemispheric dominance.

Proper writing positions should be stressed. Lined paper should be used and the child's writing samples should be retained so that he can see the progress made.

There are many currently published materials which are very helpful in the teaching of reading. Care must be taken in not choosing materials completely biased toward only one of the 4 methods of teaching reading mentioned above. Care must be taken in choosing materials suited to the level of mastery of the student. If one errs, he should err in having the materials too easy instead of too difficult.

A constant re-evaluation should be made of the child's progress in reading and writing. As the child achieves an early third grade level in reading, spelling is introduced. Early spelling should involve the ability to read and to know the meaning of the word. Early spelling mastery should be a rote learning process wherein the child memorizes the word. Following a mastery of at least 100 spelling words by rote, spelling rules may be introduced.

A great error made in the field of remedial teaching is the tendency to continue it after it is no longer necessary. The objective of the remedial teacher is to place the child in the normal and independent learning situation as quickly as possible. As soon as the child can survive on his own in his own classroom situation, he should be placed on his own and remedial teaching should stop. The classroom teacher can then complete the task in the normal classroom situation most effectively.

The same is true for speech therapy. As soon as the child has mastered enough speech to survive with his peers, the therapy should cease and the child should be placed in the situation of learning while interacting normally with his peers.

Chapter 9

CASE MATERIALS

THE AUTHOR PRESENTS these materials as illustrative of the cases he is now treating. These materials have been chosen because they are illustrative of the various kinds of problems which are met in the field of speech and reading. They are presented to help to clarify the concept and techniques of neurological organization and are not presented as a statistical justification of the concept.

From our cases of the past three years we collected a group of thirty-one children who met the following criteria:

1. Normal class in school although grade retardation was present.
2. No known neurological pathology.
3. Failure with at least one of the following: at least eighteen months of psychotherapy or at least eighteen months of remedial reading, encompassing at least three hours per week.
4. Discontinuation of all treatment other than neurological organization.
5. At least three years retardation in reading.
6. A completion of at least a five month period of neurological organization.

These children were considered failures in terms of reading by their schools and their parents.

We evaluated these children and taught them with their parents a program of neurological organization related to the areas of disorganization found during the evaluation. Each child followed treatment procedures described above as they related to his specific areas of neurological disorganization. This program was followed for forty-five minutes daily. The author re-evaluated each child at six week intervals and, on the basis of progress or the lack of progress, modified the program.

Each child followed his normal school activities and attended classes in the usual manner. The only change was the cessation of all therapy, the cessation of all tutoring and the institution of a program of activity aimed at enhancing neurological organization.

These children made a mean gain in reading of 1.8 school years in the five month period. The median gain was 1.4 and the range of gain was eight months to four years in the five month period.

SUMMER PROGRAM

We evaluated the reading progress made in a five week summer session conducted by the author. We evaluated the results of all children who attended for the past ten summers.

These children were having various degrees of difficulty with reading and 196 of the 248 total group were referred by their local schools.

The 248 children who attended the summer reading clinic during the years 1952-1962 were tested before and after the session on different forms of the Gates Reading Survey, which tests Reading Speed, Accuracy, Comprehension and Vocabulary.

The summer sessions included three and one-half hours of practice in developing neurological organization and being taught reading skills. Coupled with this was a daily swim period of an hour.

The 248 children made a mean gain in reading of 1.6 years during the five week period. The range was 4.5 years of growth to no growth. The median gain made by the 248 children was 1.4 years.

DIAGNOSIS

In an effort to ascertain the diagnostic reliability of the criteria of neurological organization we conducted the following study.

We taught twelve classroom teachers how to use the criteria in a four hour orientation session. They were taught how to evaluate the following areas: Overall coordination, homolateral crawling pattern, cross-pattern creeping, bilateral manual competence, attention span, musical aptitude, general coordination, handedness, footedness, and the predominant eye.

They were helped in collecting the data by the school nurse who administered the Keystone Visual Survey, the physical education instructor who helped to evaluate creeping and crawling, and the music teacher who evaluated musical performance.

The I. Q. range of the group was 96 to 149 and the age range was from six to thirteen.

On the basis of the teacher evaluation of neurological organization, the sections were placed in rank order from the most organized child in each section to the least organized in each section. If there was any question as to this order, on the basis of the criteria, the teacher was required to make the final placement.

Following this evaluation the children were all administered the Stanford Achievement Test appropriate to their grade level. The children in each section were placed in rank order, based on the average of their reading comprehension, vocabulary and spelling scores.

The following correlations were found when we matched teachers' evaluations of neurological organization and Stanford Achievement Test Scores:

    1. + .72
    2. + .87
    3. + .81
    4. + .64
    5. + .84

INCIDENCE

In *The Treatment and Prevention of Reading Problems* the author stated that as high as 70 per cent of poor readers had a lack of neurological organization which was observable through some confusion in laterality. There are no definitive studies which have ascertained the percentage of the total population in which some hand-eye confusion exists.

The author's good friend, retired Marine General George Van Orden, has conducted such a study in the Marine Corps during the past 11 years. General Van Orden has made the data from this extensive study available to the author.

General Van Orden's study included 38,430 cases. His cases included 1700 officer candidates, 3200 Marine reservists, 950 F.B.I. agents, and 5700 Marines immediately before combat. The remainder of the 38,430 were Marine regulars who were receiving marksmanship training.

He found that fifteen per cent of this group, or well over 5000, exhibited some confusion. They were either right handed and left eyed or left handed and right eyed. He further found that this group required a disproportionate amount of time in orientation and training to achieve the results achieved by the other 85 per cent.

BEHAVIOR

We evaluated forty-six normal children in grades three to ten who were in the proper grade for their age and who had no significant learning disabilities. No child was more than nine months retarded in reading, spelling or arithmetic, as measured by school tests.

These 46 children had in common the fact that they were behavior problems, as diagnosed by their parents and two of the three previous teachers when compared with the other children in their groups.

We evaluated these children in terms of neurological organization and found that thirty-seven of the forty-six had indications of a lack of organization.

In each case we took the next child in alphabetical order in the classroom and used that child as a control, if he was not considered a behavior problem by the teacher. If he were, we took the next child in alphabetical order as the control. We evaluated this randomly-chosen control group in terms of neurological organization and we found that only twelve of them had indications of faulty organization, as compared with thirty-seven of those exhibiting behavior problems.

STUTTERING

Stuttering is a most dramatic result of the lack of neurological organization and the lack of the complete establishment of cortical hemispheric dominance. We evaluated eighteen stutterers who had stuttered through early childhood. There were fourteen men and four women, ranging in age from eighteen to sixty-three. We found the following:

1. They not only stuttered in speech, they also stuttered (hesitated) in many other areas.

When asked to perform a task they were prone to hesitate in beginning the task. They seemed unsure of themselves when asked to perform a new, although simple, task. This was especially true in areas of mobility and vision. One, for example, had been the Captain of his High School Gym team but could not cross-pattern creep and physically stuttered (hesitated) when he started any mobility function, such as walking.

2. They all appeared to be somewhat incoordinate, but not dramatically so.

They reported that they were not particularly good athletes. As a group, they walked safely but not smoothly. Eight of them had played football in High School or College. Football is basically a bilateral sport. Not one of them had made the baseball team in High School or College. Baseball is basically a one-sided sport.

3. None of them could be classified as both an excellent reader and an excellent speller. Although most of them were bright (there were 2 Ph.D.'s and eight others were college graduates) none reported a higher verbal performance than mathematical performance on either the aptitude or achievement tests given by the College Entrance Examination Board. Every one had a higher mathematical score than verbal score, excepting for two of the women on whom we had no scores.

4. Not one of them could read over 550 words per minute with 85 per cent comprehension.

5. Not one of them earned his living through verbal activity, such as writing or teaching. Ten earned their living in mathematics, chemistry and/or science. Three did not work.

6. Eleven of them had alternating vision. This group seemed to stutter in seeing, that is, they alternated from one eye to the other in binocular vision. Seven had never been diagnosed as alternators prior to this evaluation.

7. Not one of them could stutter when singing. Each was asked to sing a familiar song on four separate occasions. Each was asked to try to stutter during their second two tries at singing. Not once did one of the stutterers stutter while singing.

8. They all had voices with good tonality and all but two enjoyed listening to music. Twelve of them had been in some group activity requiring singing during the previour five years. Eleven of them owned high fidelity record players and every one of this group had collections of classical music albums. Ten of them listened to music routinely while having meals at home. Of the two who did not enjoy music, one sang well and the other could barely carry a tune.

9. None of them could whisper without considerable difficulty. They all tended to tonalize their whispers. The one who found it least difficult to whisper could do so perfectly after five minutes of instruction. The one who found it most difficult could not do so after two hours of instruction.

10. Ten of the eighteen could not cross-pattern creep smoothly and accurately, when asked to do so initially.

11. Every one of them had some divergence in neurological organization at either a sub-cortical, cortical or dominance level. These ranged from the inability to creep properly to some mixture in sidedness.

A STUTTERER

Boy B was a perfectly normal boy of eight. He was in the middle of his group academically. His speech was normal and his arithmetic scores were slightly higher than were his reading scores at the end of the second grade. He was left handed at the time. We have no idea of other laterality factors at that time.

During the summer between second and third grades he had an accident in which his left eye was severely lacerated. The vision in the left eye was diminished to the point that only light and dark outline perception was possible.

Boy B began to stutter at the beginning of the third grade. He also began having difficulty with reading. His marks went down continuously for the next two years. His stuttering increased to the point that it was a severe and constant stutter. He also developed a divergent strabismus in the left eye because of lack of use. He received eight months of psycho-therapy and had two years of speech therapy. He was brought to the author because of the stuttering, at the end of the 5th grade.

He presented these problems: stuttering, poor reading and the divergent strabismus. The eye had been harmed structurally so that there was no hope for an improvement in vision.

We had no diagnostic alternative but to make Boy B completely right sided. We instituted a sub-cortical program at the outset upon which we planned to superimpose a new cortical hemispheric dominance. Boy B was taught to cross-pattern creep, cross-pattern walk, and mid-brain and cortical visual pursuit. He followed this program for six weeks.

At the end of the six week period we began to make him right sided. He was taught a right sided sleep pattern, we deleted tonality and we began to use the Leavell Materials on the Stereo Reader. He was also taught right sided athletic skills and he was oriented in right sidedness for all of his activities of daily living. This was followed for a period of six weeks.

At the end of this period there was a noticeable improvement in speech. There was a greater speech flow and a decrease in the stuttering. His speech, however, became fraught with reversals during this period.

As the stuttering begins to become less severe one notes, in many cases, that the speech pattern begins to change. It is not uncommon to see in the child who has almost overcome the stuttering, or in the child who has just overcome stuttering, a tendency to reverse words in speech. Such a child will say "Nutwal" for "Walnut" or "Pat" for "Tap." Such reversals are the indications that the child has returned to the normal ontogenetic path toward the development of speech, which is followed by all children. Both the phenomenon of stuttering and word reversals are considered normal in the two to three and one-half year old child. This is easily explained from a neurological basis because, at this age the beginnings of the lateralization process are being initiated. As the children experiment with laterality choices they tend to be quite ambivalent cortically, hence the development of a developmental stutter.

Boy B's family moved away during the fourth month of total treatment. Seven months after the initiating of the program Boy B's mother wrote to the author that the stutter had disappeared, reading was improving slowly but Boy B was continuing having difficulty with penmanship and spelling.

SUB-DOMINANT EYE

Boy L. was referred to the Clinic because of a visual suppression problem. Boy L. was well organized neurologically. He was completely right sided. He was so right sided that he completely suppressed the use of his left eye and, as a result, had no binocularity. The suppression was so complete that there was virtually a complete lack of function in the left eye. As a result, he was an excellent achiever but was gradually harming his left eye through lack of use.

The decision was made to attempt to retrain the left eye, but all such attempts failed. It was decided to occlude the right eye in an effort to salvage visual function for the left eye and to establish binocularity. The natural partial result of this procedure would be to disorganize the child.

We apprised the parents of the possibility of disorganizing the child but it was felt that the visual problem was acute, hence, the decision was made to try the therapy.

The predominant eye (right) was occluded for two hours per day.

Here are the Stanford Achievement Test Reading Scores:

October	6.1
February	7.2
March	8.8

We now interjected three months of occluding the predominant eye and then re-tested him in May.

May	5.6

As the child's predominant eye became less predominant, his reading ability decreased.

BRAIN INJURED

Boy C—Age 9, (WISC) I. Q. 92.

Boy C was a relatively mild athetoid. All of his symptoms of injury were at the mid-brain level and the injury was probably the result of a hypoxia suffered during a long and difficult birth.

He was in a special school for retarded children because while he was able to walk, although poorly; he was not able to learn. His walking was quite safe, but was very poor cosmetically.

He had received two years of psychotherapy without helping his reading problem. He was fairly well adjusted when we evaluated him.

Boy C presented the following problems: Not learning in special school, poor coordination, drooling, bi-lateral strabismus, and all of the coordinational lacks of the mid-brain injured child, of which the athetoid is typical. His slow, halting speech was also typical of the athetoid.

He had not established any laterality. His only accomplishment in the school was his love of music. As a result, he was put in charge of the moving and placing of chairs for all assembly programs at school.

We placed him on the following program in these successive stages:

First Month of Program
1. Homolateral crawling.
2. Auditory training at level of pons.

3. Visual training at level of pons (bi-ocular).
4. Much singing.

Second Through Sixth Month of Program
1. Cross-pattern creeping—one hour per day.
2. Auditory training and music at mid-brain level.
3. Binocular visual pursuit.
4. Cross-pattern walking.
5. New bi-lateral sports activities.

At the end of the first six months of the program we found the following changes:

1. Much improved coordination.
2. The development of binocularity (it was fragile, however).
3. More cosmetic walking.
4. Increased speech flow and increased speed in speech.
5. No significant improvement in writing, reading or spelling.
6. A trend toward left sidedness.

Although the trend toward left sidedness was not decisive, it was our opinion that he should be made completely left sided. For the next four months we followed this program:

1. All left sidedness.
2. Left sided sleep pattern.
3. Left handed skills were taught.
4. Left footed sports skills were taught.
5. We trained the left eye to be predominant, with occlusion and filtering.
6. Deletion of tonality.
7. We spent ten minutes per day going back to the sub-cortical program followed previously. This ten minutes was used as a review of those skills.

At the end of this period we found that:

1. Walking was quite normal.
2. Speech flow was normal.
3. Reading had improved dramatically. He was tested at 4.1.

4. Handwriting had improved significantly.

5. Spelling was unimproved.

We had one major setback at this point, in that Boy C had developed a convergent strabismus in his right eye.

This was probably the result of our treatment. We had superimposed a somewhat monocular task upon a fragile binocularity. We continued the entire program, excepting for the visual training. We placed him on the Stereo-Reader with a control line drawn on the right side of the reading guide. As a result, we were assured of binocular function even though we were training the left eye.

At the end of the first year of treatment Boy C was totally left sided. His coordination fitted into the lower section of the normal range. His reading level matched his chronological level. His handwriting was normal and his spelling was fair. His vision was normal.

We decided to take him out of the special school and to place him in a normal public school class. His local school accepted him. He did well academically and physically but failed socially. He was most unhappy at his new school. We removed him from the normal public school and replaced him in his former special school. During the remainder of the school year we continued a program of establishing complete dominance. In addition, we had him become a member of the Scouts, join his church group, and join an art class in his neighborhood. We insisted that he take a bus each Saturday morning and spend the day in a nearby city seeing the sights, seeing museums, going to the movies or just looking around. At the end of the school year we stopped the program completely. We sent him off to an overnight camp for boys. He adjusted to the camping nicely. He continued to improve his coordinational skills during his stay at camp.

In the fall we evaluated him and found an I. Q. of 112 on the (WISC). We placed him in the sixth grade in the public school of the next community where he was not known. He succeeded well in all areas. He scores at the 42 percentile in their population, enjoys school, has friends, and most important of all is competing with normal children in a normal class successfully.

READING RETARDATION

Boy H. Age 8½—2nd grade.

Boy H was brought to the author because he was unable to read and because he was a severe behavior problem.

He had been formerly diagnosed as brain injured, mentally retarded (I. Q. 85) and emotionally disturbed by three different clinics. Institutional care was recommended by one clinic.

Boy H was disorganized neurologically at both cortical and sub-cortical levels. His attention span was extremely short and he was very resistant to guidance.

We programmed Boy H sub-cortically with only fair success. He would not cooperate with his parents in carrying out the program. He was also excluded from his public school, as a result of his behavior. We helped to place Boy H in another school during the spring months. His behavior remained the same and he could not read.

We entered Boy H in our summer clinic and began a sub-cortical program. He mastered crawling easily and cross-pattern creeping with difficulty. He learned to cross-pattern walk easily.

As he mastered these activities his general hyperactivity decreased and he seemed to become more relaxed. There was no significant change in his reading.

He returned to school in the third grade, in the fall, and was found by his teachers to be much calmer and much more coordinate. During this school year we began a program of establishing cortical hemispheric dominance.

Although he was fairly right handed, he was both left footed and left eyed. We had great difficulty in teaching him proper head and paper positions and head to paper distance. We used filtering to train a predominant eye at reading distance and we used daily occlusion for one-half hour of viewing television. We deleted tonality and also taught him new athletic skills, using his right side, stressing the use of his right foot.

By the end of the school year he had mastered reading to a 2.5 grade level. Although he had made progress, he was still one year behind his group. He was still somewhat hyperactive but was no longer hostile.

We re-entered him into the summer program. We instituted the following program:

1. All right sidedness.
2. Right sided sleep pattern.
3. Cross-pattern creeping—twenty minutes per day.
4. Cross-pattern walking—ten minutes per day.
5. Retraining of the right eye through filtering at near-point, and occlusion at far-point—one-half hour per day.
6. Deletion of tonality.
7. Visual pursuit (cortical level only).
8. This was supplemented by the teaching of reading by various teachers of the staff.

Boy H achieved a reading score of 4.2 at the end of the summer program. His behavior and attitudes were normal for his age.

We discharged Boy H to his former public school from which he had been excluded one and one-half years previously. He adjusted well to his former school during the first few months of school. We asked the school to have him evaluated by the diagnostic clinic which had previously evaluated him. In that evaluation Boy H achieved an I. Q. on the Stanford-Binet of 133.

His performance throughout the year was excellent. He was in the top reading group in his class throughout the year. He ended the school year with a reading grade level score of 6.2. He was also elected to his school student council.

The author wishes to mention that this is by no means a typical case history. It is one of our most dramatic successes. It is included because of the possible harmful affect which could have been the result of the parents accepting any one of the three original diagnoses, brain injury, mental retardation, emotional disturbance with recommended institutional care. As one evaluates children with problems of learning, one must attempt to see through the obvious symptoms. Boy H certainly gave evidence of mental retardation by his gross inability to learn but, in reality, his I. Q. turned out to be 133. He gave evidence of being diffusely brain injured at the outset by his hyperactivity and his poor coordination at the cortical level, but he now plays football and baseball and writes and reads extremely well. He gave evidence at the outset of being emotionally disturbed, but this was obviously a *symptom* of his disability, not the *cause*. When we removed the cause, the disability in learning disappeared and the emotional problems also disappeared.

DELAYED SPEECH

Boy V. Age 4½.

Boy V was brought to the clinic because he had only six words at the age of four and one-half. He was a hyperactive and inattentive child who was daily becoming more difficult to control. His general lack of cooperation was a greater problem to his parents than was his lack of speech. His EEG indicated diffuse bilateral cortical dysfunction.

We found Boy V most uncooperative, hence, we were unable to give him any psychological tests. By observing him, we found evidence of disorganization at mid-brain and cortical levels. Because of his complete lack of cooperation, we instituted the following modified program:

1. Masking. We generally reserve this technique for more severely brain injured.[1]

2. One-half hour per day of cross-pattern creeping. This was supervised by an athletic instructor and it was completed under great duress and with many tears.

3. A weekly play therapy session aimed at helping the child to accept the discipline required during the creeping.

4. Binocular visual pursuit and a cortical program aimed at strengthening binocular skills.

5. Total deletion of music from the environment.

At the end of six weeks there was no progress. There was a trend toward right sidedness in hand use, but in no other area. We placed Boy V on a completely right sided program in addition to the above.

---

[1]For a complete description of this technique, see Delacato, C. H.: *The Treatment and Prevention of Reading Problems*, Springfield, Thomas, 1959.

At the end of the 4th month of treatment Boy V was much calmer and much more cooperative. He spoke 47 different words during the evaluation.

He then entered kindergarten and succeeded socially and emotionally. He lagged behind his classmates in the development of reading readiness. The lateralizing program continued throughout kindergarten. Both the sub-cortical program and the play therapy were discontinued. His speech, by the middle of the kindergarten year, was composed of an unlimited number of words.

At the end of the kindergarten year he scored at the 38 percentile on the Metropolitan Reading Readiness Test. He is now in the first grade with normal speech, normal behavior and is reading with the middle reading group. The only remaining area of weakness is handwriting.

STRABISMUS

Boy B, age 8, 2nd grade, (WISC) 138, Reading Level 2.2, right handed for all activities, piano lessons since age six. Problems presented by parents were poor reading progress, poor and belabored handwriting, and blindness in the right eye with a severe strabismus. This latter problem was very severe cosmetically for, in addition to having the eye turned into the nose, the size of the eyeball was much less than the size of left eye and there was a drooping of the eyelid over the right eye. The parents felt that this was more significant than were his school problems.

Sub-cortically the child was poorly organized. He had no sleep pattern and could not walk or creep in a smooth cross-pattern. He obviously had no binocularity.

We instituted the following program for the first six weeks of the pre-remedial program.

    1. Crawling practice ten minutes per day.
    2. Right sided sleep pattern.
    3. Visual pursuit at the level of pons. This included visual pursuit by his left eye of a target held in Boy B's left hand and the pursuit of a target held in his right

hand by his right eye for four minutes per day.
While each eye pursued, the other was occluded.

4. Cross-pattern creeping (mid-brain) 45 minutes per day.

5. Visual pursuit at the mid-brain level. Following a target held in his right hand with both eyes in concert four minutes per day.

6. Visual pursuit at the cortical level. Following a target binocularly. The target was held and moved about by his mother.

7. Deletion of tonality from the environment, including music lessons.

8. Right sidedness in hand and foot use.

At the end of a six-week pre-remedial period Boy B was re-evaluated. His right eye had grown so that it was barely discernable that it was smaller than the left. The (ptosis) drooping of the right eyelid had disappeared and the right eye was much straighter than it had ever been. We did not re-evaluate sight at this point.

Because of the dramatic success in such a short period it was decided to continue the pre-remedial program for another twelve week period.

When Boy B returned in twelve weeks, the eyes were the same size and they were straight. The right eye did not turn in unless it was covered for at least one minute while the left was seeing. The parents were delighted with the elimination of the strabismus.

There was, however, one problem. As the eye became straight Boy B's reading performance began to become worse. We evaluated the vision in the right eye and found that, from no vision it had now developed vision up to 20/100.

We next placed the child on the following program:

1. All right sidedness.

2. Right sided sleep pattern.

3. Delete tonality.

4. Continue binocular visual pursuit for five minutes per day.

     5. Informal practice at varying accommodation distances.

     6. Stereo-Reader practice for three ten-minute periods per day.

This program was followed for twelve weeks.

At the re-evaluation, we found:

     1. No strabismus.

     2. Both eyes the same size.

     3. Complete right sidedness, except for visual control which was still mixed.

     4. Reading level 3.4. This represented a growth of 1.2 school years during the six month pre-remedial program.

During the past four years we have treated 287 children with strabismus. These children were treated primarily for their mobility problems. They were treated secondarily for their problem of strabismus. The procedures used were those described above, aimed at enhancing neurological organization. We have successfully overcome the strabismus in 204 of these patients.

UNIVERSAL APPLICATION

There always arises the question when a new concept or procedure is used as to the universality of its applicability. If the research, or procedures, cannot be duplicated we tend to question the possible influence of the promulgator of the concept. We find those who feel that the procedures are secondary to the personality of the therapist in securing growth.

The author feels that these procedures have universal applicability and that the concepts and procedures are productive of results, and not the author's personality. The following study was conducted by Gayle L. Piper in 1962. The author has never met Mrs. Piper. The only contact which they have had is that Mrs. Piper read *The Treatment and Prevention of Reading Problems* and heard the author give a two hour lecture at Arizona State University in January, 1962.

This unpublished study is reprinted here in part. The tables and individual statistics have not been included. The study was entitled by Mrs. Piper, "Results of a Twelve-week Therapy Program in Neurological Organization and Dominant Laterality" in the Special Education Department of Mingus Union High School, in Jerome, Arizona. It is reprinted by permission of Gayle L. Piper, who conducted the study, and Keith A. West, Superintendent of Schools, Jerome, Arizona.

PROBLEM

"This testing and therapy program developed as the result of a need to find a way to help the students in the Special Education Program at Mingus Union High School bring their efforts to more normal realization.

PROCEDURES USED

"Finding a method to relieve frustrating learning experiences has long been a dream of those charged with the education of academically limited students. It has led educators down one blind alley of failure and into another. Dr. Carl H. Delacato of the Chestnut Hill Clinic in Philadelphia, Pennsylvania joined the fruitless search, and for a time traveled the usual path. But the ending this time was different.

"At a reading conference held at Arizona State University in Tempe, Dr. Delacato spoke of success. After years of research, he was experiencing success in the area of language by establishing neurological organization and dominant laterality in non-readers.

"The research resulting in this neuropsychological rationale of neurological organization and dominant laterality was begun by Dr. Carl H. Delacato in 1952 and continued by him under the direction of Dr. Temple Fay, an eminent neurosurgeon, from 1953-1956. Those three years enabled Dr. Delacato to initiate the experimental therapy for the treatment and prevention of reading problems through the avenue of neurological organization and dominant laterality. Since 1956, this neuropsychological approach to language function has benefited more than 1,500 persons with varying degrees of reading and learning problems.

"Here was a new approach. It had been tested and was proving effective. Perhaps this would help our students. As quickly as possible, these clinical methods were adapted for public school, classroom use and followed as closely as possible in the testing and therapy program in the Special Education Department at Mingus Union High School.

"The following tests were used:

1. Wechsler Scales, both Wechsler Intelligence Scale for Children (WISC), and Wechsler Adult Intelligence Scale (WAIS).
2. Gates Basic Reading Tests, Form 1, Form 2, and Form 3.
3. Tests for Neurological Organization and Laterality; i.e.,
    a. Neurological Organization—tests for sleep patterns, and cross-walking.
    b. Laterality—tests for footedness, handedness, sighting eye, and controlling eye.

"The following therapy was initiated:

1. Neurological Organization.
    a. A sleep pattern for each student's dominant laterality was taught, encouraged, and checked for progress weekly with the student.
    b. Cross-walking was taught and practiced in all special education classes a minimum of 15 minutes daily.
2. Laterality.
    a. First six-week period.
        1) Footedness and handedness for each student's dominant laterality was taught and encouraged.
    b. Second six-week period.
        1) Footedness for each student's dominant laterality was encouraged and checked.
        2) Eye dominance was reinforced by the sub-dominant eye of each student being occluded during the special education classes each day.
        3) Dominant handedness was reinforced by the sub-dominant arm of each student being tied down to the body during the special education classes each day.
3. Duration
    This therapy was begun during the last week of January, 1962, and continued through the remainder of the school year.

"Following is a record of the results obtained through the use of this therapy for the twelve-week period from February 1, 1962 through May 1, 1962, together with the interpretation and comments, for each student in the Special Education Program at Mingus Union High School.

Student 1

"Testing for neurological organization and laterality during the last week of January showed evidence of neurological disorganization and lack of laterality. Approximately six weeks after beginning therapy, this student established a moderate degree of neurological organization, laterality, and a correct sleep pattern. Coordination was improved, and a gain of .9 grade in reading achievement was made.

"During the second six week period of therapy, tests for neurological organization and laterality showed no further gain. There was evidence of greater relaxation and an obvious feeling of security with regard to motor coordination. Reading achievement showed a loss of .7 grade from the previous testing. The accuracy of this result could be questioned due to the fact that this student experienced an emotional upset just prior to testing.

"Administration of the Wechsler Intelligence Scale for Children (WISC) in September 1961 showed a Full Scale Score I. Q. of 75; this same test administered in May 1962 showed a Full Scale Score I. Q. of 90; a gain of 15 points."

Student 2

"At the time of the original testing for neurological organization and laterality, this student showed evidence of neurological disorganization. The left arm was broken and in a cast, forcing right handedness. After approximately six weeks of therapy, laterality was established, the correct sleep pattern was being maintained, coordination was improved, and there was a gain of 1.1 grades in reading achievement.

"Prior to the start of therapy, this student used right and left hands interchangeably, twisted his hair with the left hand, sustained an extremely short attention span, and chewed his tongue. These behavior deviations were no longer in evidence at the end of the first six week period of therapy.

"During the second six week period of therapy, this student again started using the right and left hands interchangeably.

Reading achievement showed a loss of 1.7 grades during this time.

"The Wechsler Intelligence Scale for Children (WISC) was administered first in September 1961 with a Full Scale Score I. Q. of 89 and again in May 1962 with a Full Scale Score I. Q. of 102; a gain of 13 points."

Student 3

"Neurological disorganization, lack of laterality, and stuttering existed at the time of the original testing. After approximately six weeks of therapy, the degree of stuttering was slightly reduced. Some success was being experienced in neurological organization, laterality, coordination, and in maintaining a correct sleep pattern. There was a gain of 1.2 grades in reading achievement.

"During the second six week period of therapy, this student began to lateralize to the left side in spite of her determined efforts to lateralize right and become a right-sided person. This student has been unable to cooperate and maintain laterality outside of the school situation. There was no gain or loss in reading achievement during this period.

"The Wechsler Intelligence Scale for Children (WISC) was administered in September 1961 with a Full Scale Score I. Q. of 75; the Wechsler Adult Intelligence Scale (WAIS) was administered in May 1962 with a Full Scale Score of 78; a gain of 3 points."

Student 4

"Neurological disorganization and lack of laterality existed at the time of the original testing. After approximately six weeks of therapy, improvement in all areas was slight. The sleep pattern was completely disorganized; there was no gain in reading achievement; no improvement in coordination. During the first six week period, this student seemed unable to put forth sufficient effort to effect improvement.

"During the second six week period of therapy, greater effort was noted. Tests for neurological organization and laterality showed little change except for some organization in the sleep pattern. There was a gain of .5 grade in reading achievement.

"The Wechsler Adult Intelligence Scale (WAIS) was administered in September 1961 with a Full Scale Score I. Q. of

74. In May 1962, this same test showed a Full Scale Score
I. Q. of 84; a gain of 10 points."

Student 5

"At the time of the original testing for neurological organization and laterality, this student evidenced neurological disorganization, lack of laterality, and both body and gait rigidity.
This could mean evidence of abnormal neuro-motor activity.
After six weeks of therapy, there was some improvement in all
areas, including motor coordination. However, sleeping three
in a small bed was not conducive to the establishment of a correct sleep pattern. A gain of .1 grade was made in reading
achievement.

"During the second six week period of therapy, there was no
apparent test gain in neurological organization and laterality
except for the recent effort to establish a correct sleep pattern.
However, body rigidity was reduced and the gait has become
more relaxed and organized. There was a gain of .4 grade in
reading achievement.

"The Wechsler Intelligence Scale for Children (WISC) was
administered in September 1961 with a Full Scale Score I. Q.
of 71. The Wechsler Adult Intelligence Scale (WAIS) was
administered in May 1962 with a Full Scale Score of I. Q. of
83; a gain of 12 points."

Student 6

"Neurological disorganization and lack of laterality was in
evidence at the time of the original testing. After six weeks
of therapy, this student was lateralized and experienced some
success in establishing a correct sleep pattern. Marked improvement in motor coordination was in evidence in the P. E.
Class. There was a .9 grade gain in reading achievement.

"During the second six week period of therapy, tests for neurological organization and laterality showed no further gain.
There was evidence of greater relaxation and freedom in body
movement and in motor organization. Reading achievement
showed a loss of .7 grade from the previous testing. The accuracy of this result could be questioned due to the fact that
this student experienced an emotional upset just prior to testing.

"Administration of the Wechsler Intelligence Scale for Children (WISC) in September 1961 showed a Full Scale Score

I. Q. of 71; this same test administered in May 1962 showed a Full Scale Score I. Q. of 91; a gain of 20 points."

Student 7

"At the time of the original testing, there was evidence of complete neurological disorganization, lack of laterality, and a rolling gait. This could mean evidence of neuro-motor disturbance. After six weeks of therapy, this student was moderately lateralized left with the exception of writing with the right hand. Neurological organization improved slightly and there was some success in establishing a correct, left sleep pattern. This student seemed unable to cooperate further at that time. The gain in reading achievement was .2 grade.

"During the last two weeks of the second six week period, this student changed handwriting from right to left. Tests showed that some neurological disorganization and lack of laterality remained. There was evidence, however, of greater cross-pattern organization. No gain or loss was made in reading achievement.

"Administration of the Wechsler Intelligence Scale for Children (WISC) in September 1961 gave a Full Scale Score I. Q. of 80; and in May 1962, a Full Scale Score I. Q. of 87; a gain of 7 points."

Student 8

"At the time of the original testing, this student evidenced neurological disorganization, lack of an established laterality pattern, walked with a severely rigid gait, and was extremely nervous. These deviations could indicate abnormal neuromotor activity. During the first six week period of therapy, this student practiced cross-walking at home and was determined to succeed in achieving a correct sleep pattern. Excellent progress was made in neurological organization and in establishing laterality. Nervousness was lessened, and this student began to walk with a relaxed, swinging gait. A gain of .8 grade was made in reading achievement.

"During the second six week period, tests for neurological organization and laterality showed little change. Although cross-pattern organization continued to be reinforced, tension increased in this student. This could have been caused by pressure from outside forces. A gain of .5 grade in reading achievement was made.

"Administration of the Wechsler Adult Intelligence scale (WAIS) in September 1961 showed a Full Scale Score I. Q. of 84; in May 1962, a Full Scale Score I. Q. of 94; a gain of 10 points."

Student 9

"At the time of the original testing, this student's behavior was characterized by hyper-activity and inattention. This condition could be of a purely traumatic etiology. There was also evidence of neurological disorganization and lack of laterality. After the first six week period of therapy, the hyper-activity was noticeably lessened, the attention span lengthened, motivation increased, and coordination improved. Moderate progress was made in neurological organization and in the establishment of a correct sleep pattern. A gain of .8 was made in reading achievement.

"During the second six week period of therapy, this student became lateralized, and had more success in establishing a correct sleep pattern. The attention span continued to lengthen and the hyper-activity to decrease. This student grew from an irresponsible child to a responsible young adult. There was a gain of .1 grade in reading achievement.

"Administration of the Wechsler Adult Intelligence Scale (WAIS) in September 1961 showed a Full Scale Score I. Q. of 84; in May 1962, a Full Scale Score I. Q. of 90; a gain of 6 points."

Student 10

"At the time of the original testing, this student evidenced such disorganization, both neurologically and laterally, that no laterality could be recommended. However, cross-walking therapy was started. After approximately four weeks of therapy, this student began to lateralize to the right side. Right laterality was encouraged and the writing hand changed from left to right. In spite of the chronological age being in the teens, this could be the change from ambidexterity to dominance which is usually experienced between the ages of six to seven, but triggered at this time by neurological organization therapy.

"This student showed body rigidity. hyper-activity, and short attention span. These deviations could be of a purely traumatic etiology.

"It was necessary to excuse this student several times during each class period for the purpose of getting a drink of water. After six weeks of therapy, this student experienced some success with neurological organization, laterality, correct sleep pattern, coordination, and the lessening of hyper-activity. He rarely asked to be excused to get a drink of water. This student is not under treatment other than the therapy in the classroom. A conclusion could be drawn that this therapy may be normalizing the cerebro-spinal canal activities.

"There appeared to be fair improvement in all areas except reading achievement. Here a loss of .5 grade was experienced. There were evident indications that another six weeks of therapy might bring improvement.

"During the second six week period of therapy, all gains were retained. Cross-pattern organization increased, and motor activity became less rigid. A gain of .2 grade was made in reading achievement.

"Administration of the Wechsler Intelligence Scale for Children (WISC) in September 1961 showed a Full Scale Score I. Q. of 67; in May 1962, a Full Scale Score I. Q. of 71; a gain of 4 points.

Student 11

"At the time of the original testing, this student evidenced neurological disorganization, lack of directionality, but seeming laterality to the right. After six weeks of therapy, there was little improvement in neurological organization, the sleep pattern remained disorganized, there was some improvement in motor coordination, and the gain in reading achievement was .3 grade. During the time of this therapy, this student experienced a health problem, and there was a confused home situation. This could be the cause for non-improvement.

"During the second six week period of therapy, neurological organization improved but laterality remained confused especially in the sleep pattern. There was a loss of .2 grade in reading achievement. Lack of directionality, as it pertains to reading and spelling, was greatly reduced.

"Administration of the Wechsler Adult Intelligence Scale (WAIS) in September 1961 showed a Full Scale Score I. Q. of 88; in May 1962, a Full Scale Score I. Q. of 97; a gain of 9 points.

Student 12

"At the time of the original testing, this student gave evidence of neurological disorganization and lack of laterality. At the end of six weeks of therapy, neurological organization was just beginning, there was moderate success in the establishment of laterality, slight success with a correct sleep pattern, and a loss of .1 grade in reading achievement. However, excellent progress in motor coordination was reported from the P. E. class.

"During the second six week period of therapy, cross-pattern organization was reinforced, and a correct sleep pattern established. There was a gain of .5 in reading achievement.

"Administration of the Wechsler Adult Intelligence Scale (WAIS) in September 1961 showed a Full Scale Score I. Q. of 77; in May 1962, a Full Scale Score I. Q. of 83; a gain of 6 points."

Student 13

"This student evidenced neurological disorganization, lack of laterality, and walked with a rigid gait at the time of the original testing. These deviations could indicate abnormal neuro-motor activity. After six weeks of therapy, some progress was made in all areas. However, the attention span remained short, the sleep pattern disorganized, and the gait was more or less as rigid as before therapy. There was a loss of .2 grade in reading achievement.

"During the second six week period of therapy, some progress was made in cross-pattern organization, but the sleep pattern remained disorganized. There was a .1 gain in reading achievement.

"Administration of the Wechsler Intelligence Scale for Children (WISC) in September 1961 showed a Full Scale Score I. Q. of 75; in May 1962, a Full Scale Score I. Q. of 80; a gain of 5 points."

Student 14

"At the time of the original testing, this student evidenced neurological disorganization, lack of laterality, and walked with a slightly rigid gait. This condition could indicate abnormal neuro-motor activity. After six weeks of therapy, excellent progress was made in neurological organization, laterality was established, and there was some success in maintaining a cor-

rect sleep pattern. Coordination improved and the walk became less rigid. A gain of 1.2 grades was made in reading
achievement.

"During the second six week period of therapy, a loss was
experienced in both neurological organization and laterality.
There was a loss of .7 grade in reading achievement.

"Administration of the Wechsler Intelligence Scale for Children (WISC) in September 1961 showed a Full Scale Score
I. Q. of 75. The Wechsler Adult Intelligence Scale (WAIS)
given in May 1962 showed a Full Scale Score I. Q. of 84; a gain
of 9 points."

WECHSLER INTELLIGENCE SCALE

September 1961 - May 1962

"Number of students differing 3 points or more on the two ad-
ministrations of the Wechsler Intelligence Scale.

Verbal Tests	Gain	Loss
Information	..	..
Comprehension	6	1
Arithmetic	4	
Similarities	4	
Vocabulary	3	
Digit Span	4	
Performance Tests		
Picture Completion		2
Picture Arrangement	5	1
Block Design	6	1
Object Assembly	3	
Coding—Digit Symbol	1	
Mazes	2	1
Verbal Score I. Q.	11	1
Performance Score I. Q.	11	1
Full Scale Score I. Q.	14	

CONCLUSIONS

"That the following tests be retained and used to evaluate
future progress of the therapy program to establish neurological
organization and dominant laterality in academically limited
students.

1. Wechsler Scales

In addition to furnishing an I. Q. Score, these tests are established as basic psychological diagnostic instruments with an SEm of ± 3, and will fall within the obtained range of two times out of three. The only deterring factor to the use of these tests is the fact that they must be used by someone trained in their administration and interpretation.

At the beginning of the school year, each student in the Special Education Department was given a Wechsler. After the twelve week period of therapy for the establishment of neurological organization and dominant laterality, these same students were again given a Wechsler. Every student had made a gain in their Wechsler Full Scale Score I. Q.'s. The gains ranged from 3-20 points as follows:

Number of Students	Point Gains
1	20
1	15
2	12
2	10
1	9
1	7
2	6
1	5
1	4
2	3

These gains have not been tested for statistical significance.

"Before therapy, the Wechsler Full Scale Score I. Q.'s ranged from 67-89; after therapy, from 71-102, as follows:

September 1961		May 1962	
Number of Students	*I. Q.*	*Number of Students*	*I. Q.*
1	89	1	102
1	88	1	97
2	84	1	94
1	80	1	91
1	77	2	90
4	75	1	87
1	74	1	84

2	71	2	83
1	67	1	80
		2	78
		1	71
Median	75	Median	84
Mean	72	Mean	86

2. Gates Basic Reading Tests (Revised)

This test seemed acceptable as a survey instrument. Its five tests give a comprehensive picture of reading achievement. The material in the five parts was considered as partially overlapping. However, as the test was used, this feature was not objectionable.

At the end of the first six week period of therapy, seven students out of the fourteen tested showed significant gains in reading achievement on the Gates Basic Reading Tests as follows:

Number of Students	Grade Gains
2	1.2
1	1.1
2	.9
2	.8

These students also showed improvement in neurological organization and in their ability to establish a degree of dominant laterality as interpreted on their individual records.

The students showing little gain, no gain, or sustaining a loss, showed comparable inability to improve their neurological organization and to establish a degree of dominant laterality as interpreted on their individual records.

At the end of the second six week period of therapy, gains in reading achievement on the Gates Basic Reading Tests were as follows:

Number of Students	Grade Gains
3	.5
1	.4
1	.2
2	.1

These students were able to maintain their gains both in neurological organization and dominant laterality. However, no new gains were apparent.

The remainder of the students found that they were unable to hold the correct sleep pattern, or that they lapsed into some form of bilaterality as noted on their individual records.

3. **Tests for Neurological Organization and Dominant Laterality**

Before starting this therapy program, tests for neurological organization and lateral dominance showed that disorganization and lack of dominance existed in the case of every student in the Special Education Program. Steps were taken at once to follow the recommendations of Dr. Delacato. Cross-walking with head turned toward the extended arm was initiated during the last fifteen minutes of each period. Apparently this cross-walking initiated and strengthened a trend toward lateral dominance. As soon as this trend became apparent, through observation and continued testing for laterality, correction for dominance was established by teaching the correct sleep pattern and the correct use of the dominant side.

At the beginning of the second six week period of this program, dominant eye and hand reinforcement was added to the existing therapy. During the special education classes, the sub-dominant eye of each student was occluded, and the sub-dominant arm of each student was tied down to his side.

The success or failure of each student to establish neurological organization and dominant laterality is noted on his individual record.

RECOMMENDATIONS

"It is recommended that this program of therapy, including testing for neurological organization and dominant laterality, be continued in the special education classes during the coming school year. Also, that a Gates Reading Survey Test be given in September and again in May to determine progress, or lack of it, in the area of language during the second year of the therapy program.

After the present twelve week period of therapy, neurological organization and dominant laterality has not been firmly estab-

lished with each student in the program. Further research will
be necessary to determine the length of time necessary to continue such a therapy program in order to obtain maximum
results."

Note: Tests were again administered at the beginning of the
Fall term. It is interesting to see what effect a three
months summer vacation had on the reading abilities of
the student. Investigation has shown that little or no
therapy took place during the summer vacation but significant gains were made by approximately 87% of the
group.

GATES BASIC READING TESTS

	Form No.1	Form No. 2	Form No. 3	Form No. 4	
Student No.	2-1-62	3-15-62	5-1-62	9-6-62	Gain - Loss
1	3.9	4.8	4.1	4.9	1.0
2	5.8	6.9	5.2	7.0	1.2
3	3.1	4.3	4.3	5.0	1.9
4	5.7	5.7	6.2	6.9	1.2
5	6.3	6.4	6.8	8.2	1.9
6	4.3	5.2	4.5	5.0	.7
7	5.7	5.9	5.9	7.0	1.3
8	7.0	7.8	8.3	8.7	1.7
9	4.9	5.7	5.8	6.1	1.2
10	3.4	2.9	3.1	3.6	.2
11	3.5	3.8	3.6	Transferred	
12	5.1	5.0	5.5	6.7	1.6
13	6.9	6.7	6.8	6.8	-.1*
14	5.4	6.6	5.9	7.1	1.7

*Emotional problem at home during past several weeks. Stu-
dent ran away from home and was returned by authorities.

Another typical study completed and sent to the author was
made by John Dunn, El Dorado School, West Covina, California
in 1961-1962. The several charts of the study are not included
below. They may be procured from Mr. Dunn, since the data is
not published.

This study, aimed at ascertaining the common factors of disability, was entitled "A Study of A Class Problem."

"The purpose of this study and report is multiple. First to be determined is can the classroom teacher objectively find the underlying problems of the individual child in preparation of constructive educational activity? Second is to find what these children have as common factors in relation to the individual type problem.

"The tests used as source information are the C.T.M.M. short form, and the C.A.T. for norms in arithmetic, reading, language and spelling.

"Vision screening is done by the school nurse with the use of a Snellen chart and the teacher or reading consultant used the Keystone Telebinocular.

"Hyperactive has reference to excessive noise, walking about the room, frequent trips to the drinking fountain, excessive toilet visits, and disturbing others trying to work in the classroom.

"Strong music background included only those children who were practicing voice or instrument lessons.

"Abnormal creeping; a deviation from the normal developmental pattern as outlined by C. H. Delacato.

"The class is a heterogenous grouping of nine boys and eighteen girls in the fifth grade with an average C.A. of ten years and an I. Q. spread from 79 to 136. The class is similar to any number of classes that have been able to build a reputation in a school as the problem group. In this class of twenty-seven children, thirteen were given neurological developmental activity in the form of developing a normal sleeping pattern, cross-pattern creeping and walking, stereo-reader work and physical development program including hand-eye coordination games.

"Positive results were observed in each case, however, pre-test and post test are not included in this report because all children were not given the test.

"The individuals are indicated by a given number and M (male) or F (female).

"The conclusions drawn from this study are limited by the number of cases involved, but are in line with theory and practice as presented by C. H. Delacato.

Mr. Dunn compared a group of normal children free of problems with a problem group. Here are some of his findings:

1. Some mixture of hand-eye-foot function (normal group 21%, problem group 70%).
2. Reading below the 50 percentile, as measured by the C.A.T. (normal group 0%, problem group 54%).
3. Spelling below the 50 percentile, as measured by the C.A.T. (normal group 7%, problem group 62%).
4. Visual acuity problems (normal group 29%, problem group 32%).
5. Poor handwriting (normal group 2%, problem group 63%).
6. Very musical (normal group 22%, problem group 43%).
7. Abnormal creeping development (normal group 2%, problem group 85%).

SPEED READING

Evelyn Wood, through the Reading Dynamics Institute, has made our nation conscious of the great variations in reading speed which exist in our schools and with adults. There are those who read more than 5,000 words per minute with good comprehension. Such readers have existed in the past and have always puzzled reading specialists.

Reading at such speeds is based upon a number of factors. There is the psychological phenomenon called "Eidetic Imagery." This phenomenon, generally known as photographic memory, is very prevalent with five and six year old children. As children begin school and as they are taught to see in parts this imagery disappears in all but a very few children. We tend to "teach it out of them" via sensitizing them to look for different types of visual factors instead of total recall in their perceptions. As a result, they lose their ability to see in wholes and to accurately reconstruct details of their visual experiences.

We now have a national reading rate of between 300 and 400 words per minute. Since this is the national average, speeds in the thousands of words per minute seem unbelievable.

The one real problem which faces us with these uncommonly high reading speeds is the fact that we have a relatively low percentage of success in teaching it to those who have made a habit of reading at what is presently considered a normal rate.

When one evaluates the speed reading programs, one finds that they are usually carried out through the use of mechanical devices which force the subject to read more rapidly. One also finds that the greatest and most universal obstacle encountered by the teachers of speed reading is *sub-vocalization*. This is the partial vocalization or tonalization of words as they are read. The subject tends to *say* the words which he is reading. The most difficult aspect about teaching subjects to read at these unbelievable speeds, while maintaining good comprehension, is that it can be achieved with only a small percentage of people.

The author made a study of six subjects who read with a speed of 1,000 to 2,000 words per minute and who, upon being tested on the material read, comprehended and retained at least 70 per cent of the material read and found the following:

1. They were relatively bright, none having an I. Q. on the Wechsler of under 120.
2. They were extremely well organized neurologically, having good sub-cortical and cortical organization. They also had good laterality right up to a good dominant-sub-dominant visual configuration. None of them were outstanding athletes.
3. They were visually oriented, in that more of their learning was done through the eyes than through the ears.
4. They were non-tonal as a group. They could not sing well and did not enjoy singing. Two of them enjoyed listening to classical music.
5. They tended to rely on sub-cortical organization to reenforce their attention. Each of them had been taught or had devised some method of involving their own hand in cueing the eyes toward greater speed. They all tended to trace a finger or their hand down over the page preceding the eyes. The hand was moved down the page almost as if *leading* the eye down the page.

Since these factors of perception, speed, general neurological organization, tonality, and sub-cortical organization are all related to overall neurological organization, we decided to investigate the possibility of predicting success with speed reading and the possibility of increasing the percentage of people with whom we succeed in teaching speed reading through a program of neurological organization.

We conducted the following study with nine boys ranging in age from thirteen to seventeen. They were chosen on the basis of neurological organization.

1-2-3—Totally right sided and well organized.

4-5-6—Totally left sided and well organized.

7-8-9—Well organized up to the level of cortical hemispheric dominance, but with confusion at the level of laterality. Each of these three boys were matched for I. Q., grade, age and general school performance level.

We were able to achieve success with three of the first six in speed reading mastery in a six week period. The criteria for success was the ability to read more than 1,500 words per minute at 80 per cent or above comprehension. The three consisted of one totally left sided and two totally right sided students.

We were not able to achieve a success with any of the boys who were disorganized at the level of cortical hemispheric dominance.

VERBAL APTITUDE

Reading, writing, speaking and listening all make up our ability to communicate. The most important aggregate measure of these abilities in the lives of students today is the *Scholastic Aptitude Test of the College Entrance Examination Board.* This is increasingly true since the crowded condition of college has become such a great educational problem.

This test is given in two areas: *Verbal Aptitude and Mathematical Aptitude.* In combination, they represent scholastic aptitude. The Verbal Aptitude score is the most important single criterion for acceptance into college. This is made even more important with the greatly increased competition for admission into college since World War II.

Two questions naturally arise at this point:

1. If optimum neurological organization is productive of better language skills with those who have difficulty with language we should be able to achieve added growths with the mildly disorganized student who doesn't have difficulty but who, nonetheless, does not achieve up to capacity.
2. If we are dealing with basic elements of the communication skills, the very aptitude in that area should be improved in addition to daily verbal performance.

We set up the following set of circumstances to assess the effect of neurological organization upon verbal aptitude. We chose as the before-and-after tests the Verbal Aptitude section of the Scholastic Aptitude Test of the College Entrance Examination Board, because:

1. It is very carefully constructed and validated.
2. It is the least affected by teaching.
3. It is so universally used and understood.
4. It is the most important single measure of verbal aptitude facing our college bound students.

As our subjects we chose an all-boys private school where all students were in a college preparatory course. We chose a small homogenous school where all the boys would receive the same teaching and the same program. The entire class consisted of twenty-five college bound boys in their Junior year, who were all required to take the College Board Entrance Examination.

The group took the Scholastic Aptitude Test administered by the College Entrance Examination Board. The 16 boys who made the highest scores in Verbal Aptitude were set off as the non-treated group. Their mean score was 547.4 points. The nine boys who made the lowest scores were set off as the experimental group. Their mean score was 397.7.

The total educational program was exactly the same for both groups. The only difference between the two groups was that the experimental group was taken out of study hall for one-half hour per day for a six week period. Each boy in the experimental group was diagnosed and was taught to follow a program of neurological organization for one-half hour per day without supervision for a six week period.

The program was set up at the outset of the six weeks and varied according to individual needs from creeping to visual training in order to establish a predominant eye. The only other difference between the control group and experimental group was that the experimental group decreased the amount of music to which it listened.

The entire group was retested by the College Entrance Examination Board.

Here are the results:

Non-treated group of sixteen boys (Mean Scores)

First Score   547.4
Re-test Score   554.2
──────
Average Gain   6.8 points

Experimental Group of 9 boys (Mean Scores)

First Score   397.7
Re-test Score   463.5
──────
Average Gain   65.8 points

The experimental group made ten times as much gain as did the non-treated group.

One boy in the experimental group made only a 2 point gain. The program was extended for an additional six weeks during the following summer, while he was not being taught at school, and ostensibly while he was on vacation. Following the added six weeks of neurological organization, he was retested by the College Entrance Examination Board. His verbal aptitude score improved by 100 points.

We must now ask the following:

Even though the ratio of growth is 10 to 1 in favor of the treated group, perhaps they would have grown just as much without the program since they were the lowest nine in the class and had the greatest distance to grow.

The question of a control group arises at this point. We did not match the groups because of the great importance to each boy of the test scores. We felt that it would not be ethical to possibly sacrifice the opportunity to go to college for a group of boys merely for the sake of purity of experimental design.

Since it was a homogeneous school and since the teaching situation was stable and competent, we went back into the school records for the previous year to see what the lowest nine boys in verbal aptitude did during that year.

The lowest nine boys of the previous year did not receive the program but received the same excellent calibre English instruction. They made an average gain of -19 points between the first and second tests, which were taken seven months apart. *That is, between the first and second tests the lowest nine boys, lost 171 points, coming to an average loss of -19 points per boy.*

Since, in educational parlance, "aptitude" and "intelligence" are interchanged, some might assume at this point that we had raised the I.Q.'s of the experimental group. This is not the case. What we did was to give them an increased ability to express their I.Q.'s (which they had all the time) more efficiently and, hence, their scores increased.

The same is true for those many children who, following a program of neurological organization, achieve higher scores on Intelligence Tests, such as the Wechsler Intelligence Scale for Children and the Stanford-Binet.

What we do to the child via improved neurological organization is to make his receptive abilities more efficient. These are visual, auditory and, to a degree, tactile and kinaesthetic. Secondly, we give him a more efficient ability to express himself via mobility, manual competence and speech. Intelligence tests attempt to measure intelligence via these modalities. For example, the Coding Test on Wechsler (which is used as a diagnostic test by many psychometrists) is based on visual perception, visual motor accuracy and speed. All of these are improved via a program of neurological organization, hence, a child does better at them. We have not changed his basic endowment, however; we have changed his ability to use his endowment. If we analyze both the Wechsler Intelligence Scale for Children and the Stanford-Binet, we find that all of the sub-tests are influenced by neurological organization or the lack of neurological organization, hence of necessity the child receives a higher score on these tests as a result of greater neurological organization.

PREVENTION

Our century's greatest contribution to the advancement of man has been the contribution in the area of communication. We have advanced our technology, we have conquered the atom, time and space as a result of our increased communication abilities. We now have so much data that needs to be processed and communicated that we have moved into the age of the giant computer to aid us in gathering, assessing, processing, storing, transporting and communicating our knowledge. These great strides in dealing with knowledge, going so far as even teaching it mechanically with our new teaching machines, have made increasingly evident the great paradox which faces us.

Although we now have mechanical devices which help us to move about our planet at incredible speeds, which can fly us to outer space, which control atomic reactions, which process our data for us, which translate such data from one language to another; we still have 40 million Americans who have not developed to their true potential one or more of the following areas of communication: speaking, listening, writing, spelling or reading.

Our concern with this problem becomes increasingly evident as we note the great efforts expended by all nations in searching out the answers to our human communication needs. We have gone into our educational systems, we have looked critically at our teachers, we revise our books, we invent teaching machines, we constantly experiment—all in an effort to increase the human ability to speak, read and write.

Happily, the new trend is toward seeking basic causes. We have exhausted the fruitless search into technique and method. This search is now reduced to the manipulation of minutiae. The public has become impatient with this search.

The author feels strongly that the search must center upon the development of the child and not upon the development of systems of teaching. As we learn more about the development and function of the nervous system, we will become better able to overcome the problems of communication.

Our research is by no means complete. As we become able to predict language problems more reliably, as we become able to diagnose them more validly, and as we treat them more successfully, we are moving toward the next significant stage—that of preventing language problems more intelligently.

BIBLIOGRAPHY

Akelatis, A. J.: A study of gnosis, praxia and language following section of corpus callosum and anterior commissure. *J. Neurosurg.*, *1*:99-102, 1944.

Akelatis, A. J.: Studies on the corpus callosum, VII, study of language function (tactile and visual lexia and graphia) unilaterally following section of the corpus callosum. *J. Neuropath. & Neurol.*, 2:226-262, 1943.

Akelatis, A. J.: Studies on the corpus callosum II, the higher visual functions in each homonymous field following complete section of the corpus callosum. *Arch. Neurol. & Psychiat.*, 45:788-796, 1941.

Alema, G. and Donini, G.: Sulle modificazioni cliniche ed elettroen cefalografiche da introduzione intracarotidea di so-amil-etil-bar-biturato di sodio nell'uomo. *Bull. Soc. Ital. Biol. Sper.*, 36:900-904, 1960.

Alexander, Peter: Radiation—imitation chemicals. *Scientific American*, July, 1959.

Anderson, A. L.: The effect of laterality localization of focal brain lesions on Wechsler-Bellevue subtests. *J. Clin. Psychol.*, 7:149-153, 1951.

Bateman, F.: On aphasia and the localization of the faculty of speech. *Med. Times and Gaz.*, pp. 486-488; 540-542, 1869.

Bates, D. R. (Ed.): *The Earth and Its Atmosphere*. New York, Basic Books, Inc., 1957.

Bender, L.: Specific reading disability as a maturational lag. *Bull. Orton Soc.*, 7:9-18, 1951.

Bibby, Geoffrey: *The Testimony of the Spade*. New York, Alfred Knopf, Inc., 1956.

Blake, M. E.: Fellow American Academy in Rome, Personal Communication, 1961.

Blau, A.: *The Master Hand*. New York., The American Orthopsychiatric Association, Inc., 1946, 5, pp. 1-206.

Brain, W. R.: Aphasia, apraxia and agnosia, in Wilson, K., *Neurology*. London, Butterworth, III, pp. 1413-1483, 1955.

Brain, W. R.: Speech and handedness. *Lancet*, 2:837-842, 1945.

Bramwell, B.: on "Crossed: aphasia and the factors which go to determine whether the "Leading" or "Driving" speech-centers shall be located in the left or the right hemisphere of the brain. With notes on a case of "Crossed" aphasia (aphasia with right-sided hemiplegia) in a left handed man. *Lancet, 1*:1473-1479, 1899.

Bremer, F.: La Synergic Interhemispheric. *Strasbourg Med., 7*:553-552, 1956.

Broca, P.: *Memoirs Sur Le Cerveau de l'Homme.* Paris, C. Reinwald, 1888, pp. 1-161.

Brownell, William A.: *Research in the Decade Ahead.* Address at the Annual Banquet, American Educational Research Association, Atlantic City, New Jersey, February 15, 1960, page 3.

Burr, H. S.: *The Neural Basis of Human Behavior,* Springfield, Thomas, 1960, pp. 1-272.

Carmichael, E. A.: Hemispherectomy and the localization of function. *Lectures on the Scientific Basis of Medicine, 3,* pp. 93-103, 1954.

Clark, M. N.: *Left-handedness; Laterality Characteristics and Their Educational Implications.* London, University of London Press, 1957.

Cohn, R.: Delayed acquisition of reading and writing abilities in children. *Arch. Neurol., 4*:153-164, Feb. 1961.

Cook, E. Gordon: *Our Astonishing Atmosphere.* New York, The Dial Press, 1957.

Cruikshank, W., Bentzen, F., Ratzeburg, F., and Tannhauser, M.: *A Teaching Method for Brain-injured and Hyperactive Children.* Syracuse Univ. Press, 1961, pp. 1-576.

Dally: Observation d'aphasie avec hemiplegi gauche. *Ann. Med. Psychol. Paris, 8*:252-253, 1882.

Dart, Raymond A., and Craig, Dennis: *Adventures with the Missing Link.* New York, Harper & Bros., 1959, p. 106.

Dearborn, O. W. F.: Ocular and manual dominance in dyslexia. *Psychol. Bull., 28*:704, 1938.

Delacato, C. H.: *The Treatment and Prevention of Reading Problems.* Springfield, Thomas, 1959, pp. 1-123.

Delacato, C. H.: *Manual of Instructions, The Delacato Stereo-Reader.* Meadville, Pa., Keystone View Co., 1961, pp. 1-23.

Doman, G., Delacato, C. H., and Doman, R.: *The Doman-Delacato Developmental Profile.* Philadelphia, The Rehabilitation Center at Philadelphia, 1962.

Doman, R., Spitz, E., Zucman, E., Delacato, C. H., and Doman, G.: *A.M.A., 174*:257-262, Sept., 1960. Initial Summary, Tables, Charts, Photographs, and Bibliography of the original article are not in cluded. This article is reprinted through the permission of the American Medical Association.

Duke Elder, W. S.: *Textbook of Ophthalmology*. St. Louis, Missouri, C. V. Mosby Co., Vol. I, 1946.

Dunbar, Carl O.: *Historical Geology*. New York, John Wiley and Sons, Inc., 1949.

Eames, T. H.: Comparison of children of premature and full term birth, who fail in reading. *J. Ed. Res.*, 38:506-508, March, 1945.

Emiliani, Cesare: Ancient Temperatures. *Scientific American*, February, 1958.

Ettlinger, G., Jackson, C. F., and Zangwill, O. L.: Cerebral dominance, in sinistrals. *Brain*, 79:569-588, 1956.

Fay, T.: Origin of human movement. *Am. J. Psychiat.*, 3:644-652, March, 1955.

Fay, T.: Rehabilitation of patients with spastic paralysis. *J. Internat., Coll. Surgeons*, 22:200-203, August, 1954.

Fay, T.: The thumb as a clinical aid in diagnostic screening of paralysis. *J. A. M. A.*, 155:729-732, June, 1954.

Fink, W. H.: The dominant eye: Its clinical significance. *Arch. Ophth.*, p. 555, April, 1939.

Flint, Richard F.: *Glacial Geology and the Pleistocene Epoch*. New York, John Wiley and Sons, Inc., Second Printing, January, 1948.

Garvin, Maxwell: *People of the Reeds*. New York, Harper & Co., 1957.

Gates, A. I., and Bond, G. C.: The relationship of handedness, eye sighting and acuity dominance to reading. *J. Ed. Psychol.*, 26:3, 1936.

Gates, R. R.: *Human Genetics*. New York, MacMillan Co., 1946, Vol. II.

Gellner, L.: *A Neurophysiological Concept of Mental Retardation and its Educational Implications*. Chicago, Levensen Research Foundation, Cook County Hospital, pp. 1-44, 1959.

Gesell, A., Ilg, F., and Bullis, G.: *Vision: Its Development in Infant and Child*. New York, Paul B. Hoeber, Inc., 1959.

Gesell, A.: *First Five Years of Life*. New York, Harper & Brothers, 1940.

Getman, G.: *How to Develop Your Child's Intelligence*. Pub. by the Author, Luverne, Minn., 1959.

Goodglass, H. and Quadfasel, F. A.: Language laterality in left-handed patients. *Brain*, 77:521-548, 1954.

Harmon, D. B.: *Notes on a Dynamic Theory of Vision*. Pub. by the author, Austin, Texas, 1958.

Hebb, D. O.: *The Organization of Behavior*. New York, John Wiley & Sons, 1949, pp. 1-319.

Hockett, C. F.: The Origin of Speech. *Scientific American, 203*:89-96, Sept., 1960.

Hooten: *Why Men Behave like Apes and Vice-Versa*. Princeton, New Jersey, Princeton University Press, 1941.

Jackson, J. H.: Defect of intellectual expression (aphasia) with left hemiplegia. *Lancet, 1*:457, 1868.

Jackson, J. H.: Observations on the physiology of language. *London, Med. Times & Gaz., 2*:275; Reprinted in *Brain, 38*:59-64, 1915.

Jensen, B. T.: Left-right orientation in profile drawing. *Am. J. Psychol., LXV*:80-83, Jan. 1952.

Jensen, B. T.: Reading habits and left-right orientation in profile drawing by Japanese children. *Am. J. Psychol., LXV*:306-307, April, 1952.

Jervis, G. A., and others: Revascularization of the brain in mental defectives. *Neurology, 3*:871-878, Dec., 1953.

Kawi, A. A., and Pasamanick, B.: Association of factors of pregnancy with reading disorders in children. *J.A.M.A., 166*:1420-1423, 1958.

Keiner, C. B. J.:*New Viewpoints on the Origin of Squint*. A Clinical and Statistical Study on its Nature, Cause and Therapy. The Hague, Martinus Nijhoff Co., 1951, pp. 1-222.

Kephart, N.: *The Slow Learner in The Classroom*. Columbus, Ohio, Charles E. Merrill Co., 1-292, 1960.

Krynauw, R. A.: Infantile hemiplegia treated by removing one cerebral hemisphere, *J. Neurol. & Psychiat., 34*:243-267, 1935.

Lashley, K. S., *Brain Mechanisms and Intelligence: A Quantitative Study of Injuries to the Brain*. Chicago, University of Chicago Press, 1929.

Lashley, K. S.: *The Problem of Serial Order in Behavior*, The Hixon Symposium (L. A. Jeffress, Ed). New York, John Wiley Sons, 1951, pp. 112-135.

Meyers, R. C.: Corpus callosum and interhemispheric communication; enduring memory effects. *Fed. Proc., 16*:298, 1957.

Meyers, R. C.: Function of corpus callosum in interocular transfer. *Brain, 79*:358-363, 1956.

Meyers, R. C.: Interocular transfer of pattern discrimination in cats following section of crossed optic fibers. *J. Comp., Physiol. Psychol.,* 48:470-473, 1955.

Money, J.: *Reading Disability, Progress and Research Needs in Dyslexia.* Baltimore, John Hopkins Press, 1962, pp. 1-222.

Newman, P.: The question of mirror-imaging in human one-egg twins. *Human Biol.,* 12:21, 1940.

Orton, S. T.: *Reading, Writing and Speech Problems in Children.* New York, W. W. Norton Co., 1937, pp. 1-215.

Penfield, W., and Rasmussen, T.: *The Cerebral Cortex of Man.* New York, The MacMillan Co., 1950, pp. 1-235.

Penfield, W. and Roberts, L.: *Speech and Brain Mechanisms.* Princeton, New Jersey, Princeton University Press, 1959, pp. 1-286.

Perria, L., Rosadini, G., and Rossi, F.: Determination of side of cerebral dominance with amobarbital. *Arch. Neurol.,* 4:173-181, Feb., 1961.

Plass, Gilbert N.: Carbon dioxide and climate. *Scientific American,* July, 1959.

Rambusch, N.: *Learning How to Learn.* Baltimore, Md., Helicon Press, 1962, pp. 1-180.

Scheidman, G.: A simple test for ocular dominance. *Am. J. Psychol.,* 43:1931.

Sherrington, C. S.: *The Brain and Its Mechanisms.* London, Oxford University Press, 1933.

Sherrington, C. S.: *Integrative Action of the Nervous System,* New Ed. Cambridge, Cambridge Univ. Press, 1947.

Sherrington, C. S.: *Man and His Nature.* Cambridge, Cambridge Univ. Press, 1951.

Skeffington, A. M.: *Differential Diagnosis in Ocular Examination.* Chicago, Wilton Pub. Co., 1931, pp. 1-200.

Smith, K. V.: The role of the commissural systems of the cerebral cortex in the determination of handedness, eyedness and footedness in man. *J. Gen. Psychol.,* 32:39-79, 1945.

Spitz, E. B.: Subdural suppuration originating in purulent leptomeningitis. *Arch. Neurol. & Psychiat.,* 22:144-149, Feb. 1945.

Spitz, E. B., Ziff, N., Brenner, C., Dawson, C.: New absorbable material for use in neurologic and general surgery. *Science, 102:*621-622, December, 1945.

Stamm, J. S., and Sperry, R. W.: Function of corpus callosum in contralateral transfer and somesthetic discrimination in cats. *J. Comp. Physiol. Psychol.,* 50:138-143, 1957.

Terzian, H., and Cecotto, C.: Su Un Nuovo Metodo Per La Deter-minazione E Lo Studio Della Dominanza Emisferico. *Gior. Psichiat. e Neuropat., 57*:1-35, 1959.

Time Magazine: Science Section, January 11, 1960.

Veeler, S.: On the amount of external mirror-imagery in double monsters and identical twins. *Proc. Nat. Acad., Sci., 15*:839, 1929.

Wada, J., and Rasmussen, T.: Intra-carotid injection of sodium amytal for the lateralization of cerebral speech dominance. *J. Neurosurg., 17*:266-282, 1960.

Wada, J.: A new method for the determination of the side of cerebral speech dominance. A preliminary report on the intra-carotid injection of sodium amytal in man. *Med. Biol., 14*:221-222, 1949.

Walker, J.: Foetal anoxia. *J. Obst. & Gynec. Brit. Emp., 61*:162-180, April, 1954.

Walls, G. L.: Theory of ocular dominance. *Arch. Ophth., 45*:387, 1951.

Washburn, Sherwood, L.: Tools and human evolution. *Scientific American, 203*:63-75, Sept., 1960.

Weiner, N.: Cybernetics. *Scientific American,* p. 614, November, 1948.

Wright, Samson: *Applied Physiology,* 9th Ed. London, Oxford University Press, 1952.

Zangwill, O. L.: *Cerebral Dominance and its Relation to Psychological Function.* Edinburgh, Oliver and Boyd, 1960, pp. 1-31.

Zollinger, R.: Removal of the left cerebral hemisphere; Report of a case. *Arch. Neurol. & Psychiat.,* Chicago, *34*:1005-1064, 1935.

INDEX

A

Aborigines, 42
Accommodation, 56
Afferent pathways, 56
Akelatis, A. J., 19
Alema, G., 20
Ambidexterity, 42
Amphibians, 36, 38, 52
Anderson, A. L., 21
Anoxia, 21
Anthropoidea, 41
Aphasia, 9, 45, 53, 102
Aptitude
  mathematical, 11
  scholastic, 11
  verbal, 170
Argon, 32
Arithmetic, 61
Articulation, 61
  problems, 113
Ataxia, 71
Athetosis, 56, 71
Audition, 50, 51, 55, 57
  binaural, 53
  monaural, 59
Auditory
  pathway, 48
  training, 114

B

Babinsky reflex, 119
Basal ganglion lesions, 71
Bateman, F., 16
Behavior, 139
Bender, L., 21
Bentzen, F., 123
Berner, D., 93
Berner, G., 93
Bibby, G., 43
Bilateral activity, 57
Bilaterality, 56
Binaural
  hearing, 53
  sound, 87
Binocularity, 87, 130
Binocular
  reading level, 95

sighting, 94
vision, 53, 55
Biocular vision, 51, 55, 86, 107
Birth, 80
  cry, 80
Blake, M. E., 42
Blau, A., 15
Bond, G. C., 19
Bottle feeding, 108
Brain injury, 69, 123, 144
Brain, W. R., 16
Bramwell, B., 16
Breast feeding, 108
Bremer, F., 19
Brenner, C., 24
Broca, P., 15
Brownell, W., 3
Bullis, G., 18
Burr, H. S., 23

C

Cambrian period, 27
Carbon dioxide, 31, 32
Carbon monoxide, 33
Carlyle, T., 15
Carmichael, E. A., 20
Cecotto, D., 20
Cerebellar lesions, 71
Cerebellum, 38
Cerebral
  lesions, 71
  peduncles, 52
Chandrichthyes, 36
Childhood diseases, 81
Chiroscopic drawing, 129
Choral speaking, 64
Circulatory system, 39
Clark, M. N., 16
Cohn, R., 22
Colliculi, 52
Communication system, 45
Contextual learning, 133
Controlling eye, 93
Convergence, 90
Coordination, 60, 84
Corpus callosum, 19

Cortex, 19, 39, 56, 62, 87
  in animals, 22
Cortical
  convolutions, 40
  hemispheric dominance, 16, 63, 73,
                          90, 92, 122
Cosmic rays, 35
Craig, Dennis, 44
Crawling, 49, 50, 72, 75, 81, 85, 106
Creeping, 53, 54, 55, 60, 75, 81, 86
  cross-pattern, 109
Cretaceous period, 29
Cross-pattern, 37, 38, 54, 86
  serialization, 60
  walking, 57, 58, 62, 88, 113
Cross-patterning, 28
Cruikshank, W., 123
Cybernetics, 23

D

Dart, R., 44
Darwin, C., 26
Dawson, C., 24
Dearborn, O. W. F., 20
Decussation, 48
Delacato, C. H., 7, 11, 24, 45, 52, 63,
            66, 69, 83, 91, 100, 130, 149,
                                 153, 167
Delayed speech, 9, 149
Development
  human, 59
  visual, 111
Developmental
  opportunity, 66, 69, 105
  progression, 68
  readiness, 60
  reading, 131
Devonian period, 28
Dinosaur, 30
Dirty hand, 42
Disease, Parkinson, 56
Diseases
  ataxia, 71
  childhood, 81
Diving, 121
Doman, G., 24, 52, 69
Doman, R., 24, 52, 69

Dominance
  cortical hemispheric, 122
  hemispheric, 14
Dominant foot, 63
Donini, G., 20
Drawing, chiroscopic, 129
Duke-Elder, W. C., 52
Dunbar, C. O., 29

E

Eames, T. H., 21
Ear, 59
Early walking, 59
Early writing, 112
Eating utensils, 109, 122
Educational methods, 25
Ettlinger, G., 16
Eidetic imagery, 168
Electro-encephalogram, 65
Emiliani, C., 30
Empathy, 9
Environment, 27
Epiphysis, 38
Evaluation, 134
Evolution, 26, 27, 45
Eye
  movements, 52, 60
  sub-dominant, 143

F

Face rotation, 98
Far-point visual control, 95
Fay, T., 23, 71, 72, 118, 153
Fish, 36
Flint, R. F., 29
Focal lesions, 21
Foetus, 48, 49
Footedness, 90, 124
Foot, writing with, 14
Fovea, 40
Function, labyrinthian, 56
Functional
  neurology, 91
  vision, 94
Fusion, 90

G

Games, 116, 125, 126
Garvin M., 42

Gates, A. I., 19
Gates, R. R., 43, 64
Gellner, L., 22
Geology, 29
Gesell, A., 18, 65, 72
Gestation, 47
Gestural ability, 103
Getman, G., 18, 117
Goodglass, H., 16
Gravity, 118, 119
Greeks, 42

H

Hand
  choice, 15, 63
  preferred, 44
  use, 55
Handedness, 16, 44, 64, 90, 125
Hands, prehensile, 39
Handwriting, 11
Harmon, D. B., 18, 132
Head-paper distance, 132
Head
  movement, 11
  position, 131
  tilt, 98
Hearing, 106
  binaural, 53
  stereophonic, 57
Hebb, D. O., 23
Helium, 33
Hemiplegia, 45
Hemispherectomy, 20, 23
Hemispheric dominance, 14
Homolateral pattern, 37, 38, 50
Homolateral patterning, 72, 105
Human
  behavior, 22
  development, 59
  movement, origins of, 23
Hydrogen, 33
Hyperactivity, 65, 84, 113, 123
Hypoxia, 80

I

Ilg, F., 18
Intelligence tests, 80
Intra-carotid injection, 20
Iraq, 42

J

Jackson, C. F., 16
Jackson, J. H., 15
Jensen, B. T., 17
Jervis, G. A., 21
Jurassic period, 28

K

Kawi, A. A., 21
Kephart, N., 117, 125
Keystone Diagnostic Series, 95
Keystone Visual Survey, 95
Kiener, G. B. S., 61
Krynauw, R. A., 20

L

Labyrinthian function, 56
La chapelle man, 43
Lady of Lloyds, 43
Language
  development, 77
  problems, 88
  symbolic, 46
Languages, 57
Lashley, K. S., 22
Lateral geniculate body, 52
Laterality, 104
Learning theory, 23
Left handedness, 96
Left sidedness, 64, 122
Lemuroids, 40
Lesions
  cerebellar, 71
  cerebral, 71
  focal, 21
  mid-brain, 71
Lombrosa, 15

M

Macula, 40
Manual dexterity, 62
Manuals, 39
Materials, 134
Mathematical aptitude, 11
Mathematics, 13
Maturation, 21
Medulla, 36
Mental retardation, 22
Methane, 33

Meyers, R. C., 19
Mid-brain, 30, 38, 52, 86, 104, 109, 110
Mid-brain lesions, 71
Mississippian period, 28
Mobility, 53, 56, 62, 81, 85
Monaural tasks, 59
Money, J., 15
Monocular reading level, 95
Monocular sighting, 94
Monotones, 124
Movement, 47
  ataxia, 71
  head, 11
  pattern, 69
Music, 44, 58, 64, 112, 123
  classes, 123
  lessons, 123
Muscle tone, 47
Mylenization, 47, 53

N

Near-point
  sighting, 95
  vision, 116
Neck reflex, tonic, 48, 49, 85
Nervous system, 18
Neural physiology, 22
Neurological maturity, 14
Neurology, functional, 91
Neurosurgery, 20
Newborn, 12, 47, 49
Newman, R., 16
Nitrogen, 31
Nitrous oxide, 34

O

Obstetrical procedure, 48
Occlusion, 107, 127
Occular motor nerves, 52
Occulo-motor nuclei, 48
Olfactory lobes, 38
Ontogenesis, 47, 66
Optic chiasm, 56
Optic lobes, 38
Optometric Extension Program, 18, 60, 61, 117
Ordovician period, 27

Orton, S., 17, 25, 92
Oxygen, 30
Ozone, 31

P

Paper position, 96, 97, 98, 99, 131
Paralateral activity, 57
Parietal lobe, 56
Parkinsons Disease, 56
Pasamanick, B., 21
Patterning, 72, 75, 105
  homolateral, 72, 105
Penfield, W., 23, 53, 56
Pennsylvanian period, 28
Perceptual confusion, 85
Permian period, 28
Perria, L., 20
Phonetic analysis, 133
Phonetics, 25, 61, 113
Photosynthesis, 30
Phylogenesis, 5, 23, 27, 46
Physical education, 116
Piano, 125
Piper, G. L., 152
Pituitary, 38
Plass, G. N., 32
Plato, 15
Play activity, 115
Pleistocene period, 29
Poetry, 64
Pons, 37, 38, 48, 85, 107
Postural centers, 52
Predominant eye, 63, 90, 91, 92, 94, 128
Preferred hand, 44
Pregnancy, 21, 80
Prehensile grasp, 55
Prehensile hands, 39
Premature children, 21
Pre-remedial period, 104, 117
Prevention, 102, 174
Primates, 39, 62
Problems, language, 88
Projection fibers, 52
Prone position, 49
Propulsion, 49

Q

Quadfasel, F. A., 16
Quadruped, 53

R

Radioactivity, 34
Rambusch, N., 125
Ratzeburg, F., 123
Reading, 62, 116
  developmental, 131
  remedial, 111
  retardation, 147
  retarded, 10
  teachers, 103
Reading level, monocular, 95
Reflex
  activity, 47
  breathing, 73
  synergy, 47
Remedial reading, 111
Reptile, 38, 39
Retarded reading, 10
Retinal fibers, 52
Revascularization, 21
Reversals, 10, 143
Roberts, L., 23, 53, 56
Romans, 42
Rosadini, G., 20
Rossi, F., 20
Rasmussen, T., 20, 23

S

Salamander, 37
Scheidman, G., 19
Scholastic aptitude, 11
School programs, 111, 132
Serialization, 53
Serialized pattern, 56
Sense organs, 36
Sensory stimulation, 73
Sherrington, C. S., 22
Sidedness, 41
Sighting
  binocular, 94
  eye, 92
  monocular, 94
  near-point, 94
Silurian period, 28
Simpson, G. G., 26

Singing, 45
Skeffington, A. M., 18
Sleep, 49
  pattern, 49, 83, 124
  position, 50, 86, 105, 106
Smith, G. E., 43
Smith, K. V., 21
Sodium amytal, 20
Solar radiation, 35
Somatic cues, 56
Sound, binaural, 57
Speaking, choral, 64
Speech, 16, 44, 58
  articulation, 61
  delayed, 91, 149
  symbolic, 57
  therapy, 102
Speed reading, 168
Spelling, 11, 62
Sperry, R. W., 19
Spinal cord, 4, 36, 85
Spitz, E., 23, 24, 69
Stamm, J. S., 19
Standardized tests, 79
Standing blackboard, 125
Stereagnosis, 56, 62
Stereophonic hearing, 57
Stereopsis, 40, 59, 62, 90, 116
Stereo-Reader, 129, 130
Stone age, 42
Strabismus, 51, 60, 61, 150
Structural analysis, 133
Stuttering, 10, 46, 64, 115, 125, 140, 142
Sub-cortex, 52
Sub-dominant
  eye, 143
  hemisphere, 21, 58
Sucking, 48
Sulcus lunatus, 43
Summer program, 137
Surgery, 24
Symbolic
  language, 46
  speech, 57

T

Tannhauser, M., 123
Tarsoidea, 40

Teaching of reading, 133, 134
Telebinocular, 95
Television, 64, 112
Temperature, 30
Tertiary period, 29
Terzian, H., 20
Tonality, 45, 83
Tonal memory, 112
Tonal starvation, 123
Tonic neck reflex, 48, 49, 85
Tools, 44
Transcortical tracts, 53
Trampoline, 117, 118, 119
Trauma, 82
Triassic period, 28
Trunkal movement, 47
Twinning, 63
Two-sidedness, 56

V

Van Orden, G., 139
Veeler, S., 16
Ventriculo-jugular shunt, 23
Verbal aptitude, 170
Vertebrates, 35, 36
Vision, 19, 50, 51, 54, 59, 89, 108
    binocular, 53, 55
    biocular, 51, 55, 86, 107
    far-point, 95
    near-point, 116
Visual
    abstraction, 59
    development, 111
    fields, 89, 113

filtration, 128
imbalance, 89
mid-line, 96
pathway, 48, 56
pursuit, 52, 112
stress, 117
training, 115, 130
Volcanic dust, 34

W

Wada, S., 20
Walker, J., 21
Walls, G. L., 20
Walking, 57, 82
    cross-pattern, 57, 58, 62, 88, 113
Washburn, Sherwood L., 44
Wechsler-Bellevue Test, 21
Wechsler Intelligence scale, 80
Weiner, N., 23
West, K. A., 153
Wolf, J., 88
Wood, E., 168
Word blind, 79
Words, 57
Word sight method, 132
Wright, S., 52, 79
Writing, 62
    position, 96, 97, 98, 99

Z

Zangwill, O. K., 15, 16
Ziff, M., 24
Zollinger, R., 20
Zucman, E., 69

DATE DUE

APR 2 4			
AUG			

Demco, Inc. 38-293